USER'S GUIDE FOR THE

STRUCTURED CLINICAL INTERVIEW FOR DSM-IV AXIS I DISORDERS

SCID-I

CLINICIAN VERSION

Michael B. First, M.D.
Robert L. Spitzer, M.D.
Miriam Gibbon, M.S.W.
Janet B. W. Williams, D.S.W.

Biometrics Research Department
New York State Psychiatric Institute
Department of Psychiatry
Columbia University
New York, New York

Copyright © 1997 Michael B. First, Robert L. Spitzer, Miriam Gibbon, and Janet B. W. Williams
ALL RIGHTS RESERVED. No part of this instrument may be reproduced or transmitted in any form or by any means, electronic or mechanical, including photocopying, or by any information storage or retrieval system, without permission in writing from the publisher.

Manufactured in the United States of America on acid-free paper
00 99 98 97   4 3 2 1

American Psychiatric Press, Inc.
1400 K Street, N.W., Washington, DC   20005

ISBN   0-88048-931-6

For citation: First MB, Spitzer RL, Gibbon M, Williams JBW: User's Guide for the Structured Clinical Interview for DSM-IV Axis I Disorders—Clinician Version (SCID-CV). Washington, DC, American Psychiatric Press, 1997. Copyright © 1997 Michael B. First, Robert L. Spitzer, Miriam Gibbon, Janet B. W. Williams.

DSM-IV criteria are used with permission from American Psychiatric Association: *Diagnostic and Statistical Manual of Mental Disorders,* 4th Edition. Washington, DC, American Psychiatric Association, 1994. Copyright © 1994 American Psychiatric Association.

Available From American Psychiatric Press:

Structured Clinical Interview for DSM-IV Axis I Disorders (SCID-I)—Clinician Version,

- User's Guide (order #8931)

    The User's Guide contains detailed instructions for administering the SCID, guiding you through the interview process and demonstrating how to make accurate DSM-IV diagnoses.

- Administration Booklet (order #8932)

    The spiral-bound, reusable Administration Booklet contains the interview questions and the DSM-IV diagnostic criteria.

- Packet of five Scoresheets (order #8933)

    One-time-use Scoresheets contain the abridged DSM-IV diagnostic criteria and provide space for recording diagnostic decisions and descriptive information.

- Administration Booklet + packet of five Scoresheets (order #8934)

- User's Guide + Administration Booklet + packet of five Scoresheets (order #8935)

The **Research Version** of the SCID is available from the Biometrics Research Department at New York State Psychiatric Institute, Unit 74, 722 West 168th Street, New York, NY 10032; (212) 960-5524. Refer to the SCID User's Guide for a discussion of the differences between the Research Version and Clinician Version of the SCID.

ACKNOWLEDGMENTS

The development of the SCID was supported in part by NIMH Contract #278-83-0007(DB) and NIMH Grant #1 R01 MH40511.

Several drafts of the DSM-IV SCID were made available to a group of experienced SCIDers, who provided extremely helpful suggestions. We are especially grateful to: Laurie Arnold, Shannon Baker, Melanie M. Biggs, Nancee Blum, Dona Davies, Dorothy Dewart, David Dunnam, Lynn Gladis, Gretchen L. Haas, Leora R. Heckelman, James D. Herbert, Steve Krebaum, Janet Lavelle, Stephanie Lewis, Kathy Shores-Wilson, Diane Stegman, Suzanne Sunday, Joseph Ventura, and Jan Weissenburger.

CONTENTS

1. Introduction

The Structured Clinical Interview for DSM-IV Axis I Disorders (SCID-I) is a semistructured interview for making the major DSM-IV Axis I diagnoses (American Psychiatric Association 1994). Structured interviews have been developed to increase diagnostic reliability through standardization of the assessment process and to increase diagnostic validity by facilitating the application of the DSM-IV diagnostic criteria and by systematically probing for symptoms that might otherwise be overlooked. Although these goals are important in clinical and research settings, the complexity and lengthiness of most structured interviews have limited their use to research studies. One of our goals in developing the SCID was to produce an efficient and user-friendly instrument so that the advantages of structured interviewing could be applied in clinical settings. A recent study conducted by Basco and colleagues (Basco et al., unpublished data) that examined the potential utility of the SCID in a community mental health setting concluded that the SCID can be used to ensure a more reliable and accurate diagnosis in a community mental health clinic setting and that it may be especially worthwhile given the complex cases often found in such clinics. The study compared a SCID diagnosis (made by a psychiatric nurse) with the diagnosis resulting from the clinician's unstructured interview and found that the SCID diagnosis was more accurate and more comprehensive (using an expert-enhanced SCID diagnosis as the gold standard). More importantly, when informed of the most accurate diagnoses, clinicians altered the medical management in 50% of cases, suggesting that the diagnostic reformulations were clinically significant. The SCID-CV represents a further refinement and adaptation of the SCID to facilitate its use in clinical settings.

2. History of the SCID

The publication of DSM-III (American Psychiatric Association 1980) revolutionized psychiatry with its inclusion of specified diagnostic criteria for virtually all of the mental disorders. Before 1980 there were several sets of diagnostic criteria, such as the Feighner Criteria (Feighner et al. 1972) and the Research Diagnostic Criteria (RDC) (Spitzer et al. 1978), as well as structured interviews designed to make diagnoses according to these systems. In 1983, in anticipation of the widespread adoption of the DSM-III criteria as the standard language for describing research subjects, work started on the SCID as an instrument for making DSM-III diagnoses. The SCID incorporated several features not in previous instruments that would facilitate its use in psychiatric research, such as the inclusion of an Overview section that allows the patient to describe the development of the current episode of illness and a modular design enabling researchers to eliminate consideration of major diagnostic classes that are irrelevant to their studies.

In 1983 the National Institute of Mental Health, also recognizing the need for a clinical diagnostic assessment procedure for making DSM-III diagnoses, issued a Request for a Proposal to develop such a procedure. Based on pilot work with the SCID, a contract was awarded to further develop the instrument. In April 1985 the Biometrics Research Department received a 2-year grant to field test the SCID and to determine its reliability in several different clinical and nonclinical subject groups (Spitzer et al. 1992; Williams et al. 1992). The SCID for DSM-III-R (American Psychiatric Association 1987) was published by American Psychiatric Press, Inc., in May 1990. Work on the DSM-IV revision of the SCID began in fall 1993. Draft versions of the revision were field-tested by interested researchers during the second half of 1994. A final version of the SCID for DSM-IV (Research Version) was produced in February 1996.

3. Versions of the SCID

The SCID was originally designed to meet the needs of both researchers and clinicians. This involved making the SCID detailed enough for the research community, but still user-friendly enough for clinicians. This duality of purpose ultimately created problems for researchers because a lot of potentially useful diagnostic information (e.g., subtypes) was left out of the DSM-III-R version of the SCID to keep it from becoming too cumbersome. However, many clinicians felt that the amount of detail that was included in the SCID still rendered it too long and complex. We have (hopefully) solved this problem by splitting the SCID for DSM-IV into two versions: Clinician Version and Research Version.

3.1 Clinician Version of the SCID (SCID-CV)

The SCID-CV is designed for use in clinical settings as a way of ensuring standardized assessments. It includes a reusable Administration Booklet and a one-time-use scoresheet. The SCID-CV covers only those DSM-IV diagnoses most commonly seen in clinical practice and excludes most of the subtypes and specifiers included in the Research Version (see Section 3.2). For most of the disorders in the SCID-CV, the full diagnostic criteria are included (with corresponding interview questions). However, some disorders are included in the SCID-CV in a summarized format in which a brief description of the disorder is provided in lieu of the full criteria set (see Table 3, page 5).

The Clinician Version of the SCID can be used in at least three ways. In the first way, a clinician does his or her usual interview and then uses a portion of the SCID-CV to confirm and document a suspected DSM-IV diagnosis. For example, the clinician, hearing the patient describe what appear to be panic attacks, may use the Anxiety Disorder module of the SCID-CV to inquire about the specific DSM-IV criteria for Panic Disorder. In this instance, the SCID-CV provides the clinician not only with the actual DSM-IV criteria for Panic Disorder, but also with the SCID questions that are efficient ways of obtaining the information necessary to judge the

diagnostic criteria. In the second way, the complete SCID-CV and SCID-II (for Personality Disorders) are administered as an intake procedure, ensuring that all of the major Axis I and Axis II diagnoses are systematically evaluated. The SCID has been used in this way in hospitals and clinics by mental health professionals of varying backgrounds, including psychiatry, psychology, psychiatric social work, and psychiatric nursing. Finally, the SCID-CV can be helpful in improving the interview skills of students in the mental health professions. The SCID-CV can provide them with a repertoire of useful questions to elicit information from a patient that will be the basis for making judgments about the diagnostic criteria. Through repeated administrations of the SCID-CV, students become familiar with the DSM-IV criteria and at the same time incorporate useful questions into their interviewing repertoire.

3.2 SCID Research Version

The Research Version of the SCID is much longer than the Clinician Version because it includes ratings for a number of subtypes, severity and course specifiers, and disorders that are diagnostically useful for researchers but that may not be of general interest to clinicians. The following disorders are included in the Research Version of the SCID-I and not in the SCID-CV: Acute Stress Disorder, Minor Depressive Disorder (DSM-IV Appendix category), Mixed Anxiety Depressive Disorder (Appendix category), and Binge Eating Disorder (Appendix category). Table 1 contains those specifiers that are included only in the Research Version of the SCID-I. Some disorders that are included only in a summarized form in the SCID-CV (i.e., a brief description instead of the full diagnostic criteria) are evaluated in their entirety in the Research Version (see Table 3). Clinicians interested in the evaluation of any of these disorders or specifiers who wish to obtain a copy of the Research Version of the SCID should contact Biometrics Research at (212) 960-5524.

Table 1. Specifiers included in the Research Version of the SCID-I (but not the SCID-CV)

Bipolar I Disorder/Bipolar II Disorder	With Rapid Cycling With Seasonal Pattern With Postpartum Onset With Melancholic Features With Atypical Features With Catatonic Features
Major Depressive Disorder	With Seasonal Pattern With Postpartum Onset With Melancholic Features With Atypical Features With Catatonic Features
Dysthymic Disorder	Early Onset/Late Onset With Atypical Features
Schizophrenia	Course Specifiers
Schizoaffective Disorder	Depressive Type Bipolar Type
Schizophreniform Disorder	With/Without Good Prognostic Features
Delusional Disorder	Persecutory/Jealous/Erotomanic/Somatic/ Grandiose/Mixed Types
Brief Psychotic Disorder	With/Without Marked Stressor
Substance Dependence	With/Without Physiological Dependence Remission Specifiers
Social Phobia	Generalized Type
Specific Phobia	Animal/Natural Environment/Blood- Injection-Injury/Situational/Other Type
Obsessive-Compulsive Disorder	With Poor Insight
Anorexia Nervosa	Restricting/Binge-Eating Type
Bulimia Nervosa	Purging/Nonpurging Type

3.3 SCID-II (for Personality Disorders)

The SCID-II is for evaluating the DSM-IV Axis II Personality Disorders. Ten of them appear in the Personality Disorders section of DSM-IV; two of them (Passive-Aggressive [Negativistic] Personality Disorder and Depressive Personality Disorder) appear in Appendix B (Criteria Sets and Axes Provided for Further Study). The SCID-II is published as a separate instrument with a separate User's Guide soon to be available from American Psychiatric Press, Inc. (First et al., in press).

4. Diagnostic Coverage

The SCID-CV is divided into six relatively self-contained modules. Although the six modules are intended to be administered in sequence, the clinician may change the order (or omit a particular module) in certain circumstances. For example,

the clinician working in a substance abuse setting may want to administer the E module (Substance Use Disorders) before modules A through D. Table 2 (below) indicates the symptoms, episodes, and disorders that are included in the SCID-CV modules. For each of the disorders listed in Table 2, the diagnosis is based on the ratings of the diagnostic criteria. Some disorders are included in the SCID-CV in a summarized format only. For these disorders (listed in Table 3), a brief description (along with a reference to those pages in DSM-IV containing the diagnostic criteria) is provided in the right-hand column in place of the full diagnostic criteria set. Furthermore, the left-hand column includes a screening question (taken from the Research Version of the SCID) relevant to that disorder. If the patient answers "yes" to the screening question, the clinician should refer to the relevant criteria set in DSM-IV and follow up with his or her own additional questions.

Table 2. Diagnostic coverage of SCID-CV

Module A: *Mood Episodes*	Major Depressive Episode Manic Episode Hypomanic Episode Dysthymic Disorder Mood Disorder Due to a General Medical Condition Substance-Induced Mood Disorder
Module B: *Psychotic Symptoms*	Delusions Hallucinations Disorganized Speech and Behavior Catatonic Behavior Negative Symptoms

Module C: *Psychotic Disorders*	Schizophrenia
	    Paranoid Type
	    Catatonic Type
	    Disorganized Type
	    Undifferentiated Type
	    Residual Type
	Schizophreniform Disorder
	Schizoaffective Disorder
	Delusional Disorder
	Brief Psychotic Disorder
	Psychotic Disorder Due to a General Medical Condition
	Substance-Induced Psychotic Disorder
	Psychotic Disorder Not Otherwise Specified

Module D: *Mood Disorders*	Bipolar I Disorder Bipolar II Disorder Bipolar Disorder Not Otherwise Specified Major Depressive Disorder Depressive Disorder Not Otherwise Specified
Module E: *Substance Use Disorders*	Alcohol Dependence Alcohol Abuse Amphetamine Dependence Amphetamine Abuse Cannabis Dependence Cannabis Abuse Cocaine Dependence Cocaine Abuse Hallucinogen Dependence Hallucinogen Abuse Opioid Dependence Opioid Abuse Phencyclidine Dependence Phencyclidine Abuse Sedative/Hypnotic/Anxiolytic Dependence Sedative/Hypnotic/Anxiolytic Abuse Other or Unknown Substance Dependence Other or Unknown Substance Abuse
Module F: *Anxiety and Other Disorders*	Panic Disorder With Agoraphobia Panic Disorder Without Agoraphobia Obsessive-Compulsive Disorder Posttraumatic Stress Disorder Anxiety Disorder Due to a General Medical Condition Substance-Induced Anxiety Disorder Anxiety Disorder Not Otherwise Specified Adjustment Disorder

Table 3.   **Disorders included in Module F of the SCID-CV**
                 without diagnostic criteria

- Agoraphobia Without History of Panic Disorder
- Social Phobia
- Specific Phobia
- Generalized Anxiety Disorder
- Somatization Disorder
- Undifferentiated Somatoform Disorder
- Hypochondriasis
- Body Dysmorphic Disorder
- Anorexia Nervosa
- Bulimia Nervosa

5. Basic Features of the SCID-CV

Appropriate Subjects for the SCID. The SCID-CV may be administered to either psychiatric or general medical patients. The language and diagnostic coverage make the SCID-CV most appropriate for use with adults (age 18 or older), but with slight modification, it may be used with adolescents. Anyone with an eighth grade education should understand the language of the SCID-CV. Some individuals with severe cognitive impairment, agitation, or severe psychotic symptoms cannot be interviewed using the SCID-CV. This should be evident in the first 10 minutes of the Overview and in such a case there is no point in conducting an unnecessarily prolonged interview when accurate data are unlikely to be obtained. The SCID-CV may be used instead as a diagnostic checklist, with information obtained from other sources (see page 7 of the User's Guide).

Administration Booklet and Scoresheet. The SCID-CV uses two separate books: a reusable Administration Booklet that contains the interview questions and the DSM-IV diagnostic criteria, and a one-time-use scoresheet containing the DSM-IV diagnostic criteria (abridged) on which the clinician records his or her diagnostic decisions. During the interview, the two booklets are used side by side, with the clinician referring to the Administration Booklet for the interview questions and the diagnostic criteria while making the ratings on the Scoresheet. Space is available below each item in the Scoresheet for the clinician to record descriptive information that supports the diagnostic ratings. It should be noted that there is not a one-to-one correspondence between the pages in the Administration Booklet and the pages in the Scoresheet. Thus, clinicians do need to be sure that they are marking the correct items on the Scoresheet as they are inquiring about the symptoms while using the Administration Booklet.

Inclusion of an Overview. Before systematically inquiring about the presence or absence of particular DSM-IV criterion items, the SCID-CV begins with an open-ended Overview of the present illness and past episodes of psychopathology. This Overview provides an opportunity for the patient to describe the presenting problem in his or her own words, as well as for collecting certain types of information that may not be covered when assessing specific diagnostic criteria (e.g., prior treatment, social and occupational functioning, and the developmental context of the psychopathology). By the end of the Overview, the clinician should have gathered enough information to formulate a tentative differential diagnosis.

Diagnostic Flow. The sequence of questions in the SCID-CV is designed to approximate the differential diagnostic process of an experienced clinician. Since the DSM-IV diagnostic criteria are embedded in the SCID-CV and are assessed as the interview progresses, the interviewer is, in effect, continually testing diagnostic hypotheses. Note that for some disorders, the diagnostic criteria are not listed in the same order as in DSM-IV but have been reordered to make the SCID-CV interview more efficient or user-friendly. For example, the D criterion for Schizophrenia is listed after the A criterion to allow the interviewer to skip out of Schizophrenia immediately if the temporal relationship between psychotic and mood symptoms is not consistent with a diagnosis of Schizophrenia.

Ratings Are of Criterion Items, *Not* of Answers to Questions. Although specific structured questions are provided to help elicit diagnostic information, it is important to understand that the ratings on the SCID-CV are judgments about the diagnostic criteria and not necessarily the patient's answers to the questions. Although the majority of the SCID-CV questions can be answered by a simple "yes" or "no," more often than not an unelaborated "yes" answer is not enough information for the clinician to determine whether a criterion is met. It is usually necessary to ask the patient to elaborate or provide specific examples. For instance, one of the questions for a Major Depressive Episode asks whether the patient has had "trouble thinking or concentrating." Before rating the corresponding criterion (i.e., "diminished ability to think or concentrate . . .") as present, the clinician should ask additional questions (e.g., "what kinds of things do you have trouble concentrating on?"). A positive rating should be made only after the interviewer is satisfied that the criterion is met. Sometimes this might even entail seeking corroborating information from other sources (i.e., family members, previous records). In some cases it may be useful to read or paraphrase the wording of the criterion to make the concept clearer to the patient.

Ultimately, the clinician must make a *clinical judgment* as to whether a diagnostic criterion is met. If the clinician is convinced that a particular symptom is present, he or she should not allow the patient's denial of the symptom to go unchallenged. In rare cases an item may be coded as present even when the patient steadfastly denies it (e.g., a patient who claims that spending 2 hours a day in a hand washing ritual is not "excessive or unreasonable"). Yet, if the clinician doubts that a symptom is present even after hearing the patient describe it, the item should be rated as not present. It is not necessary to get the patient to agree that the symptom is not present.

Diagnostic Summary. When the interview is completed, the clinician indicates the DSM-IV diagnoses on the SCID-CV Diagnostic Summary. For each disorder, the clinician indicates whether it is "current" (i.e., if the full criteria have been met at any time during the current month), and/or "lifetime" (if the full criteria have ever been met during the patient's life). Certain specifiers can also be indicated by checking them off. Ratings for Axis IV (Psychosocial and Environmental Problems Checklist) and Axis V (Global Assessment of Functioning Scale) follow the scoring of the Axis I Disorders.

Sources of Information. The clinician should use all available sources of information about the patient in making the ratings. This might include referral notes and the observations of family members and friends. In some cases the clinician may need to confront the patient with discrepancies between his or her account and other sources of information.

When the patient is a poor historian (e.g., a hospitalized patient with acute psychotic symptoms and agitation, a chronic patient with cognitive impairment), much of the information may have to be drawn from the medical records. Before beginning the interview with such a patient, the clinician should review the chart, note symptoms and dates of prior hospitalizations in the Life Chart (page 12 of the Scoresheet), and record a brief description of the pertinent symptoms in the section of the SCID in which they are assessed (e.g., record psychotic symptoms in the B module). In these cases, interviewing the patient may provide relatively little additional information, and the SCID-CV will serve not so much as an interview guide, but rather as a place to record systematically symptoms that have been documented in the hospital records.

6. Administration

Ordinarily, the SCID-CV is administered in a single sitting and takes 45–90 minutes, depending on the complexity of the psychiatric history, the skill and experience of the clinician, and the ability of the patient to describe his or her psychopathology succinctly. Usually the SCID-II (for Personality Disorders) is administered following the SCID-CV, sometimes on another day. (Instructions for administering the SCID-II are contained in the SCID-II User's Guide, published separately.) With certain types of patients, the SCID-CV may have to be administered in several sittings. If additional information becomes available after the interview is completed, the SCID-CV should be modified accordingly.

7. SCID-CV Conventions and Usage

Note: When you review the next section, we recommend that you have copies of the SCID-CV Administration Booklet and Scoresheet handy.

1. *Item labels.* Each rated item in the SCID-CV has been assigned a label consisting of a letter (indicating the SCID-CV module) and a number. These labels, which appear to the left and to the right of each item in both the Administration Booklet and the Scoresheet, allow the clinician to match the interview item in the Administration Booklet with the corresponding item in the Scoresheet. Note that there is *not* a one-to-one correspondence between the pages in the Administration Booklet and the pages in the Scoresheet so that the same item label will appear on different pages in the two documents. For example, the depressed mood item for a Major Depressive Episode is labeled "A1" on page 3 of the Administration Booklet and page 13 of the Scoresheet. These labels are also used to indicate target locations for the skip-out instructions. For example, the skip-out instruction after item A2 on the bottom of page 3 in the Administration

Booklet (if there has never been a period of depressed mood or loss of interest lasting at least 2 weeks) instructs the clinician to skip to item A16 on page 8 of the Administration Booklet. There is a corresponding skip-out under the ratings for item A2 on page 13 of the Scoresheet, directing the clinician to skip to item A16 on page 15 of the Scoresheet.

2. *Two-column format for Modules A, B, E, and F.* In the Administration Booklet, Module A (Mood Episodes), Module B (Psychotic Symptoms), Module E (Substance Use Disorders), and Module F (Anxiety and Other Disorders) contain interview questions with the diagnostic criteria in a two-column format. In the left-hand column are the interview questions (in lowercase letters) and directions to the clinician (in capital letters). The right-hand column contains the DSM-IV diagnostic criteria that correspond to the interview questions.

Two-column ratings. The diagnostic ratings for the two-column format are recorded by the clinician on the right-hand column of the Scoresheet. Each criterion is rated on the Scoresheet as either "?," "–," or "+." Following is an explanation of each rating:

? = Inadequate information to code the criterion as either "–" or "+"

A "?" should be coded in situations in which there is inadequate information for a more definitive rating. For example, in rating the sleep item for Major Depressive Episode, a "?" would be appropriate for a patient who cannot remember whether sleep was disturbed during the episode. When diagnostic information is questionable, a "?" may also be given to indicate uncertainty (e.g., a patient denies hallucinations but has been observed to talk to himself in a way that suggests that he may be hearing voices).

When subsequent information makes it possible to recode the criterion, the "?" should be crossed out and the correct rating circled. Subsequent information may come from another source, or from the patient later in the same interview, or in a later interview. In some cases, however, it may never be possible to obtain the information and the item must ultimately be recoded as "–."

– = Below threshold or false

Below Threshold. The symptom described in the criterion is either absent or below the diagnostic threshold specified in the criterion (e.g., Major Depressive Episode criterion A(5) is rated "–" if there is no psychomotor retardation or agitation, or if agitation or retardation is present, but it is not severe enough to be observable by others).

False. The criterion statement is false (e.g., only one of five required symptoms is present).

+ = Threshold or true

Threshold. The threshold for the criterion is just met (e.g., patient reports being depressed for 2 weeks) or more than met (e.g., patient reports being depressed for several months).

True. The criterion statement is true (e.g., "Criteria A, B, and C are coded +").

Skip-out instructions. Skip-out instructions control the diagnostic flow of the interview, directing the clinician to jump to a different part of the SCID-CV. These skip-out instructions are contained in boxes that extend across the entire page. Depending on the content of the skip instruction, the clinician may (or may not) be instructed to skip to another item in the SCID-CV. The clinician must always look out for skip instructions. When there is no skip-out instruction, the clinician should always proceed to the next question (item).

Remember that whenever you skip ahead in the Administration Booklet, you also have to skip over the corresponding items in the Scoresheet. To facilitate this, the target item label is included in a box hanging under the "–" rating in the right-hand column of the Scoresheet. Note, however, that the page number under the item label refers to the Scoresheet rather than the Administration Booklet. For example, on page 73 of the Administration Booklet, the skip-out instruction for item F40 (criterion A(1) for Posttraumatic Stress Disorder) instructs the clinician to skip to item F65 on page 77 of the Administration Booklet if the rating for F40 is "–." According to the corresponding item, F40 at the top of page 53 of the Scoresheet, the box in the right-hand column hanging under the "–" indicates that the target item of the skip-out (i.e., F65) is located on page 56 of the Scoresheet.

There are several places in the SCID-CV where skip-out instructions are used:

- *To skip out of the evaluation of a disorder when criteria can no longer be met.* To minimize the number of questions needed to make a diagnostic assessment, skip instructions are embedded within the evaluation of a criteria set. If a particular rating makes it impossible for the criteria to be met, the clinician is instructed to skip to the evaluation of the next disorder. For example, in the Administration Booklet, the skip instruction following item F1 in Panic Disorder (on page 65 of the Administration Booklet) instructs the clinician to skip to page 70 (of the Administration Booklet) and proceed with the evaluation of Obsessive-Compulsive Disorder (starting with item F25) if the rating for item F1 is "–" (i.e., there is no need to continue with the evaluation of Panic Disorder if there are no unexpected panic attacks). In some cases (e.g., item A10), the clinician is instructed to ask the patient an additional question (e.g., "Have there been any other times when you've been depressed...?" and then skip based on the answer to that question.

- *To skip to another section when the evaluation of a disorder is completed.* For example, in the Administration Booklet, the instruction after item A29 tells the clinician to skip the evaluation of Hypomanic Episode and Dysthymic Disorder after making a rating of a Manic Episode (e.g., "YOU ARE FINISHED EVALUATING MOOD EPISODES. GO TO MODULE B (PSYCHOTIC AND ASSOCIATED SYMPTOMS), B1 (PAGE 25)." This is because the presence of a Manic Episode (most likely indicating a diagnosis of Bipolar I Disorder) automatically rules out a diagnosis of Bipolar II Disorder and Dysthymic Disorder, so there is no need to evaluate the criteria for Hypomanic Episode or Dysthymic Disorder.

- *To skip to another section if a particular condition is true.* For example, the instruction at the beginning of the evaluation of Mood Disorder Due to a General Medi-cal Condition (page 20 of the Administrative Booklet) tells the clinician to skip to the evaluation of Substance-Induced Mood Disorder if the mood symptoms are not temporally associated with a general medical condition.

3. *Decision tree format for Modules C and D.* Module C (Psychotic Disorders) and Module D (Mood Disorders) use a decision tree format. Each diagnostic criterion is contained in a box with two outgoing arrows. The clinician evaluates the criterion in the box based on symptom information obtained in Modules A and B. In some cases, additional information may be needed to evaluate the criterion and clarifying questions are also provided. If the criterion in the box is true, the clinician should rate the item "yes" on the Scoresheet and follow the "yes" arrow in the tree. If the criterion is false, the clinician should rate the item "no" on the Scoresheet and follow the "no" arrow in the tree.

4. *Lifetime history versus current status.* The initial question for each diagnosis generally begins with "Have you ever had ...?" to prepare the patient for inquiry about a lifetime history of the disorder. Once the clinician has determined that the criteria have been met for a disorder, the section ends with a question to help the clinician determine whether the criteria have been met in the past month (e.g., "Have you had [DEPRESSIVE SYMPTOMS] in the past month?"). If the full criteria have been met in the past month, the clinician records this by checking the corresponding item in the Scoresheet (e.g., D16) and also checking the current box for the corresponding disorder in the Diagnostic Summary section of the SCID-CV (see section 9.1.1, page 14 of the User's Guide). Note that the SCID-CV does not inquire about past episodes of Dysthymic Disorder or Adjustment Disorder.

5. *Questions asked verbatim.* Questions not in parentheses are to be asked verbatim of every patient. The only exception to this basic SCID-CV rule is for those instances in which the patient has already provided the necessary information earlier in the SCID-CV interview. For example, if during the Overview the patient states that the reason for coming to the clinic is that he or she has been very depressed for the past couple of months, the clinician would not then ask verbatim the initial question in the A module: "In the last month, has there been a period of time when you were feeling depressed or down for most of the day nearly every day?" In such instances, however, the clinician should NOT just assume that the symptom is present and code the item "+" without asking for confirmation, because some aspect of the criterion may not have been adequately explored (e.g., duration). Instead, the clinician should confirm the information already obtained by paraphrasing the original question, saying, for example, "You've already told me that you were feeling depressed for the last couple of months. Was there a 2-week period in which you were depressed for most of the day, nearly every day?"

6. *Parenthetical questions*. Questions in parentheses are to be asked when necessary to clarify responses. This does not imply that the information the question is designed to elicit is any less critical. For instance, the question for the first item in a Major Depressive Episode has the inquiry "as long as 2 weeks?" in parentheses. This indicates that if the patient has already discussed the duration of the depressed mood, it is not necessary to ask if it lasted 2 weeks. However, the 2-week duration of the depressed mood is still a critical requirement for rating this symptom as "+." In addition, the clinician is encouraged to add as many of his or her own questions as needed to feel confident about the validity of the rating.

7. *"OWN WORDS."* Many of the questions contain the phrase OWN WORDS in brackets. This indicates that the clinician is to modify the question using the words of the patient to describe the particular symptom. For example, if the patient refers to a Manic Episode as "when I was wired," then the clinician might rephrase the question "Which time were you the most [high/irritable/ OWN WORDS?]" to "Which time were you the most wired?"

8. *Providing descriptive information*. The clinician is encouraged to ask the patient to provide specific details of thoughts, feelings, and behaviors to increase the validity of the criterion ratings. This information should be recorded on the SCID-CV Scoresheet (in the "notes" space provided for each criterion) to document the evidence used to justify the clinician's rating. When such information comes from charts or other in-

formants, the source should also be noted on the SCID-CV Scoresheet.

9. *Multiple clauses*. Note that some of the items consist of two or more clauses. For clauses that are joined by "OR" (e.g., alcohol is often taken in larger amounts OR over a longer period than was intended), a rating of "+" for the full item is made if EITHER of the clauses is judged to be true.

10. *Not Otherwise Specified*. The SCID-CV provides a Not Otherwise Specified (NOS) diagnosis for only the Mood, Psychotic, and Anxiety Disorders. Other cases diagnosed in DSM-IV as NOS (e.g., Eating Disorder NOS) should be classified on the Diagnostic Summary as "Other DSM-IV Axis I Disorder."

11. *Secondary Versus Primary Psychiatric*. Most of the diagnoses covered in the SCID-CV include a criterion that requires the clinician to decide whether or not the psychopathology is directly caused by a general medical condition (GMC) or substance use (i.e., "the disturbance is not due to the direct physiological effects of a substance or general medical condition"). This criterion was known as the "organic" exclusion criterion in DSM-III-R. If the clinician determines that the disturbance is caused by the direct physiological effects on the central nervous system of a general medical condition or substance use, it is considered to be a **secondary** condition. In this case, the SCID-CV directs the clinician to skip out of the diagnosis being considered and diagnose instead a Mental Disorder Due to a General Medical Condition or Substance-Induced Disorder. In contrast, if the clinician judges that a general medical condition or substance is NOT the cause of the psychopathology, then the disorder being assessed is **primary** and the clinician continues with the evaluation. For example, in evaluating the criteria for a Major Depressive Episode on page 6 (of the Administration Booklet), the clinician comes to criterion D ("not due to the direct physiological effects of a substance or a general medical condition"). If the interviewer decides that the depression is secondary to a substance (e.g., cocaine), then a diagnosis of Cocaine-Induced Mood Disorder is made. However, if the interviewer decides that the depression is primary, the interview continues on the top of page 7 (of the Administration Booklet) with criterion E.

NEOPHYTE SCIDers BEWARE: The double negative in this criterion is a common source of confusion. The exclusion criterion **IS MET** (coded +) if the disturbance is **NOT** due to a substance or general medical condition (i.e., it is primary)—say to yourself "*Yes* or TRUE ('+'), there is *no* substance or general medical condition." The criterion is **NOT MET** (coded "–") if it is **NOT TRUE** that the disturbance is not due to a substance or general medical condition (i.e., it is secondary)—say to yourself "*No* ('–'), there *is* an etiological substance or general medical condition."

There are two steps to the assessment of whether a disturbance is primary or secondary:

STEP 1: *Is there evidence that a general medical condition or a substance MAY be etiologically associated with the disturbance?* If so, further investigate the possibility that the disturbance is secondary by going on to step 2; if not (i.e., the disturbance is primary), rate the criterion "+" and go on to the next item.

Evidence that a general medical condition or substance may be associated includes: 1) the presence of a general medical condition or substance use during the disturbance; and 2) the general medical condition or substance has been reported in the research literature to cause the psychopathology. The questions provided on the left-hand side of this criterion (in the Administration Booklet) serve to establish a temporal relationship. The list of general medical conditions and substances listed below the criterion indicates those conditions and substances that are known to be associated with the psychopathology (at least according to DSM-IV). Note that this list is not exhaustive—many other conditions or medications can cause psychopathology. The clinician is encouraged to consult other clinicians or reference sources when in doubt. Once the clinician has decided that there is evidence of a possible etiological relationship, the box below the questions instructs the clinician to skip to the section of the SCID-CV where the Mental Disorder Due to a General Medical Condition or Substance-Induced Disorder is evaluated. For example, in evaluating item A12 on page 6 of the Administration Booklet, the clinician discovers that the patient has been using cocaine around

the time of the depressed mood. Since withdrawal from cocaine is known to cause depression, the clinician should skip to page 20 (in the Administration Booklet) to evaluate whether the criteria for a Cocaine-Induced Mood Disorder are met.

STEP 2: *Is there evidence for a causal relationship between the disturbance and the substance or general medical condition so that the disturbance can be considered secondary (i.e., are the criteria met for a Mental Disorder Due to a General Medical Condition or Substance-Induced Disorder)?*

The actual clinical judgment about whether the disturbance is primary or secondary is made in the context of evaluating whether the criteria are met for a Mental Disorder Due to a General Medical Condition or a Substance-Induced Disorder. (*NOTE:* For a complete review of how to decide whether a disorder is secondary, see page 25 in the User's Guide for a discussion of the criteria for Mood Disorder Due to a General Medical Condition and page 26 for a discussion of the criteria for Substance-Induced Mood Disorder— these discussions also apply to Psychotic and Anxiety Disorders due to general medical conditions or substances). After deciding whether the particular Mental Disorder Due to a General Medical Condition or Substance-Induced Disorder is present or absent, the clinician is instructed to return to the section of the SCID-CV where the "organic" exclusion criterion was being evaluated to complete the rating for that criterion. If a Mental Disorder Due to a General Medical Condition or a Substance-Induced Disorder is diagnosed and it is judged to have completely accounted for the psychopathology, then the disturbance is secondary, the "organic" criterion is rated "–" (i.e., it is NOT true that the disturbance was not due to a general medical condition or substance) and the clinician is instructed to skip out. However, if the disturbance is primary (i.e., neither a Mental Disorder Due to a General Medical Condition nor a Substance-Induced Disorder was present), then the "organic" criterion should be coded "+" (i.e., it is true that the disturbance was NOT caused by a general medical condition or substance) and the clinician should proceed to the next item.

An example may help clarify matters: the patient has recurrent unexpected panic attacks. Criterion C (Item F18) on page 67 (of the Administration Booklet) asks the clinician to consider whether the panic attacks are secondary (i.e., is a general medical condition or substance use responsible for the condition?). If the clinician were to discover that the panic attacks occur only during periods of heavy coffee use, the clinician would jump to page 81 (and then to page 83) to consider whether Caffeine-Induced Anxiety Disorder accounts for the attacks. If a diagnosis of Caffeine-Induced Anxiety Disorder is ultimately made, then, when returning to the evaluation of criterion C for Panic Disorder (item F18), the clinician would rate it as *not* present (code "–" in the Scoresheet) and skip to F25, page 70 (in the Administration Booklet), and evaluate the criteria for Obsessive-Compulsive Disorder. Otherwise, if the panic attacks are primary (i.e., in the absence of a substance or general medical condition etiology), the clinician would rate criterion C as present (code "+" in the Scoresheet) and continue with the evaluation of criterion D for Panic Disorder (item F19).

If the clinician knows from the Overview that the diagnosis is likely to be excluded because of an etiological general medical condition or substance use, he or she may skip directly to the rating of the criterion for the Mental Disorder Due to a General Medical Condition or Substance-Induced Disorder, rather than spend time documenting a syndrome that is ultimately going to be excluded on the basis of a general medical or substance etiology. For example, if the patient has described being depressed during a few months when he or she was taking steroids, the clinician may ask whether that was the only time the patient has ever been depressed. If that was the only time, the etiological general medical condition/substance criterion for Major Depressive Episode (item A12) is coded "–," and the clinician should proceed as instructed [i.e., skip to item A16, page 8 of the Administration Booklet (Manic Episode)].

12. *Consideration of treatment effects.* Symptoms should be coded as present or absent without any assumptions about what would be present if the patient were not receiving treatment. Thus, if a patient is taking a sedative every night and no longer has insomnia (initial, middle, or terminal), then the symptom of insomnia should not count toward the minimum five symptom requirement for a current Major Depressive Episode (unless the insomnia was present and persisted during the same 2 weeks as the other depressive symptoms).

13. *Clinical significance.* Most disorders in the SCID include a criterion that requires there to

be clinically significant distress or impairment before a DSM-IV diagnosis can be made. For most patients in psychiatric settings, this judgment is a non-issue because there is implied clinical significance by the fact that the person is in treatment for the disturbance. This criterion is more important (and more difficult to evaluate) in settings where the patients are not identified as "psychiatric patients" (e.g., in primary care settings). Note that there are two components to the concept of clinical significance: distress and impairment, either of which indicates clinical significance. Seeking treatment is certainly evidence of significant distress or impairment in functioning. Impairment may involve, for example, lost days at work or school or disruption of relationships.

8. SCID Dos and Don'ts

→ **DO** use the Overview to obtain the patient's perception of the problem and treatment history.

→ **DON'T** ask in the Overview for details about specific symptoms that are covered in later sections of the SCID-CV.

→ **DO** get an overview of the current illness at the beginning of the interview to understand the context in which it developed.

→ **DON'T** leave the Overview section until you have enough information to formulate a list of the diagnostic possibilities.

→ **DO** stick to the initial questions, as they are written, except for minor modifications to consider what the patient has already said, or to request elaboration or clarification.

→ **DON'T** make up your own initial questions because you feel that you have a better way of getting the same information. Your minor improvement may have a major unwanted effect on the meaning of the question. A lot of care has gone into the exact phrasing of the questions, and they work in nearly all cases.

→ **DO** ask additional clarifying questions to elicit details in the patient's own words, such as "Can you tell me about that?" or "Do you mean that . . . ?"

→ **DON'T** use the interview as a checklist or true/false test.

→ **DO** take care to ensure that the item you are rating on the Scoresheet corresponds to the question you are asking in the Administration Booklet.

→ **DON'T** skip to an item in the Administration Booklet without also skipping to the corresponding item in the Scoresheet.

→ **DO** use your judgment about a symptom, considering all of the information available, and confront the patient (gently, of course) about responses that conflict with other information.

→ **DON'T** automatically accept a patient's response if it contradicts other information or you believe it is not valid.

→ **DO** make sure that the patient understands what you are asking. It may be necessary to repeat or rephrase questions or ask patients if they understand you. In some cases it may be valuable to describe the entire syndrome you are asking about (e.g., a Manic Episode).

→ **DON'T** use words or jargon that the patient does not understand.

→ **DO** make sure that you and the patient are focusing on the same (and the appropriate) time period for each question.

→ **DON'T** assume that symptoms that a patient is describing cluster together in time unless you have clarified the time period. For example, the patient may be talking about a symptom that occurred a year ago and another symptom that appeared last week, when you want him or her to focus on symptoms that occurred jointly during a 2-week period of possible Major Depressive Episode.

→ **DO** focus on obtaining the necessary information to judge all of the particulars of the criterion under consideration. As noted earlier, this may require asking additional questions.

→ **DON'T** focus only on getting an answer to the SCID-CV question.

→ **DO** give the patient the benefit of the doubt about a questionable psychotic symptom by rating a "–."

→ **DON'T** call a subculturally accepted religious belief or an overvalued idea a delusion. DON'T confuse ruminations or obsessions with auditory hallucinations.

→ **DO** make sure that each symptom noted as present is diagnostically significant. For example, if a patient says that he has *always* had trouble sleeping, then that symptom should *not* be noted as present in the portion of the SCID-CV dealing with the diagnosis of a Major Depressive Episode (unless the sleep problem was worse during the period under review). This is particularly important when an episodic condition (such as a Major Depressive Episode) is superimposed on a chronic condition (such as Dysthymic Disorder).

→ **DO** pay attention to double negatives, especially in the exclusion criteria. For example, the phrase "is NOT better accounted for by Bereavement" means that a rating of "–" is made if it is better accounted for by Bereavement and a "+" if it is NOT.

→ **DON'T** code "–" for an exclusion criterion when what you *really* mean is that the excluded condition is NOT present. For example, if the criterion reads "NOT due to the direct physiological effects of a general medical condition or substance," then a rating of "–" means that the disturbance is secondary, i.e., due to a general medical condition or substance, and a rating of "+" means primary, i.e., NOT due to a general medical condition or substance. (Think: "Yes, we have no bananas" → '+,' we have no etiological medical condition or substance.")

→ **DO** proceed sequentially through the SCID-CV unless an instruction tells you to skip to another section.

→ **DON'T** skip a section without completing it because you feel certain that it does not apply (e.g., don't skip the psychotic symptoms section because you have no indication from the Overview that the patient has ever had any psychotic symptoms).

9. Special Instructions for Individual Modules

This section of the User's Guide provides specific instructions for each of the individual SCID-CV modules.

9.1 SCID-CV Diagnostic Summary

The Diagnostic Summary is arguably the most important single module of the SCID-CV because, in practice, it is the Diagnostic Summary that is often used as the sole source of diagnostic information. No matter how carefully the interview was done, a mistake or omission on the Diagnostic Summary will result in erroneous diagnostic data.

9.1.1 Scoring the Individual Disorders

After the interview is completed the clinician fills out the Diagnostic Summary, located at the front of the SCID-CV Scoresheet. This involves going through the Diagnostic Summary and checking the "lifetime" box if the criteria have EVER been met for the disorder, and the "current" box if the criteria have been met in the past month. Note that this process entails the clinician simply transcribing the relevant information from the section of the Scoresheet containing the rating for the item that is indicated in parentheses next to the name of the disorder—no additional clinical judgment is required. If the clinician wants to indicate a diagnosis that is not covered by the SCID-CV, it can be recorded under the "Other DSM-IV Axis I Disorders" section, which is listed after Adjustment Disorders. For those diagnoses that are made only if currently present (i.e., Dysthymic Disorder, Adjustment Disorder), only the "current" box is available.

Mood Disorder Due to a General Medical Condition, Substance-Induced Mood Disorder, Psychotic Disorder Due to a General Medical Condition, Substance-Induced Psychotic Disorder, Anxiety Disorder Due to a General Medical Condition, and Substance-Induced Anxiety Disorder include the instructions "indicate GENERAL MEDICAL CONDITION: ____" or "indicate substance: _____." The specific etiological general medical condition or substance should be noted in the space provided.

9.1.2 Scoring DSM-IV Axis IV

DSM-IV Axis IV is for noting clinically relevant psychosocial and environmental problems that may be important in the clinical management of the patient. Problem areas are presented in a checklist format to ensure a comprehensive evaluation. The clinician should check any relevant problem areas and then specify the particular type of problem (e.g., unemployment, divorce). In most cases, information gathered during the course of the SCID-CV (especially from the last section of the Overview) is sufficient for recording Axis IV. If not, additional questions should be improvised as needed (e.g., "Does your depression put a major strain on your relationship with your wife?").

9.1.3 Scoring DSM-IV Axis V

An Axis V evaluation entails rating the patient using the Global Assessment of Functioning (GAF) Scale. To make a GAF rating, the clinician chooses a single value that best reflects the patient's current overall level of functioning. The GAF scale is divided into 10 ranges. The description of each range in the GAF has two components: the first part covers symptom severity, and the second part covers functioning. The GAF rating is within a particular 10-point range if EITHER the symptom severity OR the level of functioning falls within the range. For example, the first part of the description of the range 41–50 indicates "serious symptoms (e.g., suicidal ideation, severe obsessional rituals, frequent shoplifting)" and the second part "any serious impairment in social, occupational, or school functioning (e.g., no friends, unable to keep a job)." The GAF scale is like two scales wrapped into one: a scale for measuring symptom severity and another scale for measuring the level of social and occupational functioning. Note that the SCID-CV has a provision for two GAF ratings: current (lowest level in the past month) and highest GAF score achieved in the past year (which can be helpful in indicating the patient's potential level of functioning when the current episode improves).

Four Steps to an Axis V Rating

STEP 1: Starting at the top level, evaluate each range by asking yourself, "Is EITHER the patient's symptom severity OR the patient's level of functioning worse than what is indicated in the range?"

STEP 2: Keep moving down the scale until you reach the range that best matches the patient's symptom severity OR level of functioning, WHICHEVER IS THE WORST.

STEP 3: Double check the range immediately BELOW the range you have picked in step 2. It should be too severe for BOTH symptom severity AND level of functioning. If not, you stopped too soon and should keep moving down the scale.

STEP 4: To determine the specific number within the 10-point range, consider whether the patient is functioning at the higher or lower end of the range.

An alternative method is to treat the GAF as if it were two scales: one for symptom severity and another for level of functioning. Using the steps above, make one rating for severity and a second for level of functioning. The WORST of the two can be used as the GAF score.

9.2 Overview

This section allows the clinician to obtain enough information to make a tentative differential diagnosis before inquiring systematically about specific symptoms in the later modules. The Overview in the SCID-CV begins with basic demographic data, educational history, and occupational history. Note that the questions are not listed in the Administration Booklet but appear only on the Scoresheet, with space provided next to each question for the clinician to write in the answers. These questions both help develop rapport with the patient before the more potentially difficult questions about symptomatology and may provide the first clue to the effects of past psychopathology on functioning. The remaining parts of the Overview are divided into sections covering the nature of the present illness or exacerbation and sections covering the history of prior mental illness. This division works well when the patient has a current episode of illness that is distinct from prior episodes. However, when there is a chronic disorder with periods of partial remission and exacerbation (e.g., chronic Major Depressive Disorder), the clinician must make a clinical decision about what constitutes the onset

of the current period of illness. Often this judgment will be based on information about when there was a gross change in functioning (e.g., had to quit job, dropped out of school). The sequence of questions in the Overview will not flow as smoothly if the current illness is not clearly distinguishable from chronic or recurrent problems, and the clinician may have to improvise questions to elucidate the complete clinical course.

If, when asking about a history of past treatment it becomes clear that the patient has had a particularly complicated history, it may be useful to turn to the Life Chart, located at the end of the Overview on page 12 of the Scoresheet. This chart provides a framework for recording past treatment history in a chronological fashion.

When the SCID-CV is used to interview patients with psychotic symptoms, it is often necessary to use ancillary information to elicit responses in the Overview. For example, if a patient has no chief complaint and denies having any idea of why he or she was brought to a psychiatric unit, the clinician might say: "The admission note said you were burning your clothes in the bathtub, and your mother called the police. What was that all about?" In many cases in which the patient is currently psychotic, most of the information may have to come from the chart or from other informants.

In the Overview, patients are asked about all past treatments, including medications. The clinician should be sure to question a patient about any prescribed medications that do not seem appropriate for the condition described. This often gives a clue to problems that the patient has not mentioned. For example, a patient who reports only chronic depression, but was treated with lithium in the past, may then describe a possible manic episode when asked why lithium was prescribed. (Of course, a prescribed medication should NOT be used to justify a diagnosis without documentation that the disorder actually met criteria, because medication is sometimes prescribed inappropriately.)

9.3 Module A. Mood Episodes, Dysthymic Disorder, Mood Disorder Due to a General Medical Condition, and Substance-Induced Mood Disorder

Module A begins with ratings for Major Depressive Episode, Manic Episode, and Hypomanic Episode. Please note that the ratings for those disorders that are defined by the presence (or history) of one or more of these episodes are made in later modules (i.e., Module C for Schizoaffective Disorder and Module D for Major Depressive Disorder, Bipolar I Disorder, and Bipolar II Disorder).

Ratings for Major Depressive Episode (items A1–A15)

Criterion A (items A1 and A2): Establishing the 2-Week Duration. Because of the treatment implications of diagnosing a current mood disturbance, the clinician is asked to focus first on whether the criteria are met for a Major Depressive Episode within the past month. The clinician's first task is therefore to determine whether there has been a 2-week period of depressed mood and/or loss of interest that has occurred in the past month (or had an earlier onset but persisted into the past month). If, as is often the case, depressed mood has lasted for much longer than 2 weeks, it is crucial to establish with the patient which specific 2-week period in the past month to focus on (presumably the worst 2 weeks). If the patient reports that the depressed mood has been pretty much the same for the entire month, the clinician should focus on the most recent 2 weeks. Even if there is some doubt about whether the depressed mood has lasted a full 2 weeks, the clinician should inquire about the specific symptoms anyway because it often turns out that a patient who minimizes a problem when first asked may, on further reflection, recall that he or she was, in fact, symptomatic for a full 2 weeks.

If there are no periods of depressed mood or loss of interest in the past month, the clinician should inquire about any past periods of depressed mood or loss of interest. Because of the difficulty that some patients may have in recalling specific symptoms that characterized a depressive episode occurring years earlier, the clinician should pick a specific 2-week interval during the depressive period to be the focal point for the subsequent eight questions. We recommend using holidays, seasons, or other life events (e.g., birthdays, graduation) as "landmarks" in pinpointing the 2-week period in which the depression was the worst. This process of carefully reviewing the patient's past also serves to transform the time period from an abstraction to a more vivid memory so that the reporting of specific symptoms is more likely to be valid. For ex-

ample, a patient reports being depressed for several months during his junior year in college. The clinician may try to pinpoint a 2-week interval as follows: "I know it's hard to be this precise, but I will need to focus on a 2-week period when it was the worst. Were you depressed during the fall semester of your junior year or in the spring?" Patient answers "spring," "Was it before or after spring break?" "How close was it to finals?" and so forth.

In those situations in which the patient reports more than one past episode in his or her lifetime, the clinician should establish which of the episodes was "the worst," and subsequent questions should focus on the worst 2-week period during that "worst" episode. However, there are a couple of exceptions to this rule. If there has been an episode in the past year, the clinician should ask about this period even if it was not "the worst," because it is more recent, and therefore the patient is more likely to remember details about it. Also, when there are several possible episodes, experienced SCID users may want to avoid focusing on an episode that is likely to be ruled out because of a possible etiological general medical condition or substance or because it may be better accounted for by Bereavement.

Common Pitfalls. One of the most common errors made in this section is the failure to ensure that each symptom has been present for "most of the day, nearly every day." We therefore strongly recommend that you specifically ask, "Was that true for most of the day, nearly every day, during this period?" after each symptom, even to the point of tedium, because there is no other way to ensure that this duration requirement is met. Do not assume that if the first several symptoms are present for most of the day, nearly every day, the rest will also have this pattern. Note that criterion A(9) (item A9) does not have to be present every day—recurrent suicidal ideation or a single suicide attempt alone warrants a rating of "+."

A second common pitfall is to forget to ask about the second half of an item when the patient answers "no" to the first part. For example, item A7 can be rated "+" if EITHER worthlessness OR excessive or inappropriate guilt has been present. If the patient denies feelings of worthlessness, then the clinician should NOT code the item "–" but must follow up that question with an inquiry about excessive or inappropriate guilt.

A third issue is how to count symptoms that occur in the context of a comorbid general medical condition. General medical conditions may present with the same types of symptoms as those that characterize a depressive episode (e.g., weight loss, insomnia, fatigue). Should they be attributed to the depression or the medical condition? The rule in DSM-IV is to consider such symptoms as part of the depressive episode UNLESS they are clearly attributable to the medical condition. For example, insomnia related to frequent nocturnal coughing spells in a person with bronchitis should not count for item A4. Similarly, symptoms should not count toward a Major Depressive Episode if they are better accounted for by another disorder. For example, weight loss due to refusal to eat food because of the delusion that the food is poisoned should not be rated "+."

A final issue is whether to consider as part of the depressive episode symptoms that have been present before the onset of the episode (e.g., chronic insomnia). Such symptoms count toward a diagnosis of a Major Depressive Episode only if they have become appreciably worse during the depressive episode. For example, if a patient who usually takes 30 minutes to fall asleep finds that it has been taking 2 hours to fall asleep since the episode began, it would make sense to rate item A4 as "+" for the episode.

Criterion A(1): Depressed Mood (item A1). Depressed mood may be acknowledged directly ("I've been feeling depressed") or by one of its many synonyms (sad, blue, tearful, "down in the dumps," "I can't stop crying"). Depressed mood in a Major Depressive Episode can be distinguished from "everyday" (i.e., nonpathological) depression or the "blues" only by virtue of its persistence and severity. To count toward this criterion, the patient's depressed mood must have been present for most of the day, nearly every day, for at least 2 weeks. Note that the criterion can be rated "+" based on observational information, even if it runs counter to the patient's subjective reporting (e.g., a stoic elderly patient denies being depressed whereas the staff reports that the patient has been continuously tearful).

Criterion A(2): Decreased Interest or Pleasure (item A2). Although the cardinal symptom of a Major Depressive Episode is depressed mood, it may be diagnosed in the absence of a subjective report of depression. Some patients, particularly those with severe presentations, have lost the capacity to feel sadness. Others may have a cognitive style or come from a cultural setting in which feelings of sadness are downplayed. For such patients, loss of interest or pleasure counts as a "depressive equivalent" and can be substituted for depressed mood when defining the 2-week interval that applies to criteria A(3)–A(9). Evidence of this symptom may be that the patient reports a general diminishing of pleasure (e.g., nothing makes me happy anymore) or specific examples such as no longer reading books, watching television, going to the movies, socializing with friends or family, or having sex. When rating this item, note that complete loss of interest or the inability to experience pleasure is not necessarily required for a rating of "+"—evidence that there is a significant reduction in the ability to experience pleasure will suffice.

Criterion A(3): Change in Appetite or Weight (item A3). This item should be rated "+" if there has been a significant change in appetite (either increased or decreased) OR a significant change in weight. Note that the criterion gives an example of significant weight change as at least a 5% change in body weight in a 4-week period. This example may complicate the evaluation of a Major Depressive Episode because the other criteria have to be present only over a 2-week period. In most cases, patients with a significant weight change also have a change in appetite that has occurred throughout the 2-week period. In fact, severe weight loss with only a mild decrease in appetite may suggest that a possibly undiagnosed general medical condition is causing the weight loss. Be sure to inquire whether the weight loss was intentional (i.e., a part of normal dieting or an Eating Disorder); if it was, it should not count toward the diagnosis of a Major Depressive Episode.

Criterion A(4): Sleep Disturbance (item A4). Insomnia may be manifested in many different ways, all of which can count for this item. These include difficulty falling asleep, waking up many times in the middle of the night, and awakening much earlier than is normal for that person, with an inability to fall back asleep. Hypersomnia is sleeping much more than is normal for the person. Note that it is difficult and potentially not very meaningful to establish an absolute definition of the number of hours of sleep that constitute insomnia or hypersomnia because of wide variability in individuals' need for sleep. However, sleeping

2 hours more or less than is typical on a daily basis would constitute hypersomnia or insomnia. Note that hypersomnia should not be coded for someone who stays in bed for most of the day but is not sleeping.

Criterion A(5): Agitation or Retardation (item A5). Psychomotor agitation and retardation refer to changes in motor activity and rate of thinking. While many depressed patients describe a subjective feeling of being restless or slowed down, this item should not be rated "+" unless the symptoms are visibly apparent to an outside observer (e.g., the patient is either pacing and unable to sit still or seems to move in slow motion). If the symptom is not currently present and observable by the clinician, there must be a convincing behavioral description of past agitation or retardation that was observed by others. Distinguish the feelings of being slowed down in psychomotor retardation (e.g., "I feel like I'm walking through a vat of molasses") from feelings of having no energy, which are coded in the next item.

Criterion A(6): Fatigue (item A6). Patients with this symptom may report feeling tired all the time, "running on low power," feeling "weak," or feeling totally drained after minimal physical activity. When a patient complains about not feeling like doing anything, the clinician should differentiate between lack of energy and loss of interest or motivation (item A2), which may or may not also be present.

Criterion A(7): Feelings of Worthlessness or Excessive Guilt (item A7). Be careful in rating this item because patients who are depressed, but who do not have the full syndrome of a Major Depressive Episode, often acknowledge feeling bad about themselves or feeling guilty. The actual item requires a more severe disturbance in self-perception—either feelings of *worthlessness* OR *excessive* or *inappropriate* guilt. If, after asking a patient how he or she feels about himself or herself, you get an "I feel bad" or "I don't like myself," it is often helpful to present the patient with the actual item (e.g., "How bad does that get? So bad that you feel worthless?"). Similarly, while patients often report feeling guilty about the negative impact their problems have on others ("I feel so guilty for being such a burden"), such feelings are often not excessive or inappropriate. A true positive response requires evidence

of exaggerated and inappropriate guilt (e.g, "I feel like I've ruined my family forever").

Criterion A(8): Concentration Problems or Indecisiveness (item A8). Cognitive impairment in depression is sometimes severe enough to resemble dementia. With less severe but still significant impairment, a patient may be unable to concentrate on any activity (e.g., watching TV, reading a newspaper) because of an inability to filter out brooding thoughts. Clinicians should note that the impairment caused by this symptom may vary, depending on the patient's baseline. For example, a theoretical mathematician may still be able to watch TV but no longer be able to concentrate on mathematical proofs—in such an instance, a rating of "+" would be warranted. Note that the second half of this item taps a different type of impairment (i.e., indecisiveness). A patient with this symptom may report feeling paralyzed by even simple decisions, such as which clothes to wear for the day or what to eat for lunch. A rating of "+" is made if a patient has signficant concentration problems *or* difficulty with everyday decisions.

Criterion A(9): Suicidal Ideation (item A9). This is the only symptom that does not have to be present nearly every day for at least 2 weeks to warrant a rating of "+." Any recurrent suicidal thoughts or behavior, or any single suicide attempt is sufficient, as well as frequent thoughts such as "I'd be better off dead" or "My family would be better off if I were dead." If there are current suicidal thoughts, it is imperative that the clinician explore the seriousness of these thoughts and take appropriate action.

Self-mutilating behavior (cutting, burning, etc.), without suicidal intent, that is only an expression of anger or frustration or is done with the aim of controlling anxiety is coded "–."

Criterion A(10): Check for Other Periods of Depressed Mood (item A10). If the full criteria are not met for the 2-week period identified in items A1 or A2, the clinician is instructed to consider whether there may be any *other* periods of depression that are more likely to meet the criteria for a Major Depressive Episode, before skipping to the evaluation of a Manic Episode. This question is included as a double check to make sure no other likely candidate episodes are skipped.

NOTE: Criterion B from DSM-IV, which ensures that the symptoms do not also meet the criteria for a Mixed Episode, has been omitted from the SCID because the presence of a Mixed Episode is inferred by the overlap of Major Depressive and Manic Episodes.

Criterion C: Clinical Significance (item A11). DSM-IV has added this "clinical significance" criterion to most of the disorders to emphasize the requirement that a symptom pattern must lead to impairment or distress before being considered a mental disorder. This criterion has been included in the SCID for the sake of completeness, and we imagine that it will only rarely be necessary to ask the corresponding question. This criterion may help the clinician make a decision as to whether a diagnosis should be made in studies of individuals who have not sought the help of a mental health professional, for whom the severity of the presentation may be near the symptomatic threshold for a disorder.

Criterion D: Ruling Out Direct Physiological Effects of a Substance or a General Medical Condition (item A12). This criterion instructs the clinician to consider and rule out a general medical condition or a substance as an etiological factor. See pages 10–12 (of the User's Guide) for a general discussion of how to apply this criterion and pages 24–27 (of the User's Guide) for a discussion of the criteria for Mood Disorder Due to a General Medical Condition and Substance-Induced Mood Disorder.

Criterion E: Ruling Out Simple Bereavement (item A13). At this point in the SCID-CV, a depressive period lasting at least 2 weeks has been identified. If, however, that depressive period is considered to be a normal and expectable reaction to the death of a loved one, it is not diagnosed as a Major Depressive Episode but would instead be Bereavement. Therefore, the judgment required in this item is whether the depressive reaction has crossed the line (in terms of persistence and severity) from Bereavement to Major Depressive Episode. DSM-IV provides two guidelines for diagnosing Major Depressive Episode rather than Bereavement: 1) if the depressive symptoms (i.e., at least five, most of the day, nearly every day) have persisted for at least 2 months following the loss, or 2) if certain depressive symptoms that are particularly uncharacteristic of Bereavement are present (e.g., suicidal ideation, psychomotor retardation, etc.). *Note that this is one of those double negative items; that is, a "+" is coded if it is NOT better accounted for by Bereavement ("Yes, we have NO Bereavement"), and a "−" is coded if it IS Bereavement.*

Number of Episodes (item A15). After making a rating of "+" on item A14 indicating that the criteria are met for a Major Depressive Episode, the clinician is instructed to make a rough estimate about the number of episodes. This entails asking the patient to report how many separate times he or she has had a Major Depressive Episode—it does not mean that the clinician is expected to inquire about each symptom for each episode. For most purposes, an estimate of the number of episodes will be sufficient.

Ratings for Manic Episode (items A16–A29)

The questions for Manic Episode are designed to detect lifetime episodes (i.e., "Have you ever had a period of time . . .?") because most patients being evaluated will not currently be in a Manic Episode. In cases in which the patient appears to be currently manic, rephrase the questions for the current episode (e.g., "Are you now feeling . . .?").

Criterion A(1): Elevated or Irritable Mood (item A16). This criterion requires a persistently elevated, expansive, or irritable mood. Patients often describe periods of irritability that are clearly not associated with a Manic Episode. Most commonly, such periods are either Major Depressive Episodes with irritability as an associated feature or chronic irritability that is a symptom of a personality disturbance. If there is no evidence of current or past manic mood or behavior, the clinician can skip to A45 (Dysthymic Disorder). However, if there is any question whether the irritability might be part of a Manic or Hypomanic Episode, the clinician should continue to ask all the manic questions to make a judgment as to whether the irritability is a symptom of a Manic or Hypomanic Episode or is better accounted for by another condition.

Criterion A(1): 1-Week Duration (item A17). The criteria sets for Manic and Hypomanic Episodes are symptomatically identical but differ in terms of minimum duration (Manic Episode has a minimum duration of 1 week, whereas a Hypomanic

Episode has a minimum duration of only 4 days) and severity (Manic Episodes cause significant impairment in functioning, whereas Hypomanic Episodes, by definition, must NOT cause significant impairment). If the patient acknowledges having a period of elevated or irritable mood but denies that it has lasted every day for at least a week (unless hospitalized, in which case you can make a diagnosis of Manic Episode), then the clinician is instructed to skip to A30, page 13 in the Administration Booklet, to check for a Hypomanic Episode.

Criterion B(1): Increased Self-Esteem (item A18). It is important to remember that to count a B symptom toward the diagnosis of a Manic Episode, the symptom must be persistent and clinically significant. Therefore, merely being more self-confident than usual would not suffice for a rating of "+." There must be grandiosity or inflated self-esteem that is clearly not justified by a realistic evaluation.

Criterion B(2): Less Sleep (item A19). The patient should report needing less sleep than usual (i.e., getting by on 2 (or more) hours less sleep) to justify a rating of "+" for this item. The prototypic patient feels that he or she does not need to sleep. Although some may report waking up and not feeling tired, more commonly the patient describes feeling driven or "wired" and cannot calm down enough to sleep. Note that the phrase "feels rested after only 3 hours of sleep" is included in the DSM-IV criterion only as an example and should not be misconstrued as a specific requirement for a rating of "+."

Criterion B(3): Pressured Speech (item A20). The increase in talkativeness is manifest in both the rate and amount of speech. The speech often has a driven quality, as if there is so much to say and not nearly enough time to say it. If present during the interview, it may be very difficult for the clinician to interrupt the patient's monologue.

Criterion B(4): Racing Thoughts (item A21). This criterion can be rated "+" based either on the patient's subjective report that his or her thoughts are racing OR on the clinical judgment that flight of ideas has been present (based either on observation of the patient's speech pattern or by history). Flight of ideas involves thoughts that are loosely connected, with the patient jumping from one topic to another very quickly, with only the

slightest thread of thematic connection between topics. In some cases, the connection may be based on sound rather than meaning (clang association).

Criterion B(5): Distractibility (item A22). Distractibility refers to an inability to filter out extraneous stimuli while attempting to focus on a particular task. For example, the patient may have trouble focusing on the clinician's questions because of being distracted by a police siren and may need to jump up from the interview and investigate what is happening.

Criterion B(6): Increased Activity or Agitation (item A23). As a consequence of elevated mood, increased energy, or increased self-esteem, the patient may become involved in more activities than usual. Typical "manic" activities may include calling friends at all hours of the night, writing lots of letters, or beginning new creative projects. Alternatively, the increase in activity may be more diffuse and be evident as psychomotor agitation (e.g., being unable to sit still). The presence of either an increase in activity or psychomotor agitation warrants a rating of "+."

Criterion B(7): Involvement in Pleasurable Activities (item A24). In the pursuit of pleasure, excitement, or thrills, patients may engage in activities that are uncharacteristic, without regard to possible negative consequences. Typical examples include lavishly spending large sums of money on luxury items, gifts for others, or expensive vacations, driving too fast, or engaging in reckless or unsafe sexual behavior. Note that the SCID-CV question (i.e., "Have you done anything that could have caused trouble for you or your family?") is relatively nonspecific in that it will detect any behavior that reflects poor insight or judgment. This item should be coded "+" ONLY if the behavior is inherently pleasurable. For example, problematic behavior occurring in response to a command hallucination or delusion (e.g., accosting strangers with the news that doomsday is approaching) would not warrant a rating of "+."

Criterion B: (3/4 out of 7) (item A25). Note that the number of items required to meet criterion B depends on whether criterion A was coded "+" based on euphoric mood versus irritable mood. If euphoric mood has been present, then only three B criteria need to have been present. In contrast, irritable mania requires a minimum of four items to help differentiate it from an irritable Major Depressive Episode.

If the full criteria are not met for the manic period identified in item A16, the clinician is instructed to consider whether there may be any *other* manic periods that are more likely to meet the criteria for a Manic Episode before skipping to the evaluation of Dysthymic Disorder. This question is included as a double check to make sure that no other likely candidate episodes were passed over.

NOTE: Criterion C from DSM-IV, which ensures that the symptoms do not also meet the criteria for a Mixed Episode, has been omitted from the SCID because the presence of a Mixed Episode is inferred by the overlap of Major Depressive and Manic Episodes.

Criterion D (item A26). A comparison of the criteria for Manic and Hypomanic Episodes reveals that these two entities share the same symptoms but differ on the degree of severity. As indicated in this criterion, the symptoms in a Manic Episode must be sufficiently severe to cause marked impairment, require hospitalization, or include psychotic features. Otherwise, a diagnosis of Hypomanic Episode should be considered (and in most cases, would be warranted). For this reason, if a rating of "−" is made, the clinician is instructed to skip to criterion C for Hypomanic Episode if there are no other past episodes that might have met the criteria for a Manic Episode. Note that the SCID-CV continues with Hypomanic criterion C because criteria A and B for Hypomanic Episode have already been met because they are identical to criteria A and B for Manic Episode.

Criterion E (item A27). This criterion instructs the clinician to consider and rule out a general medical condition or a substance as an etiological factor. See pages 10–12 (in the User's Guide) for a general discussion of how to apply this criterion and pages 24–27 (in the User's Guide) for a discussion of the criteria for Mood Disorder Due to a General Medical Condition and Substance-Induced Mood Disorder.

Number of Episodes (item A29). After making a rating of "+" in item A28, indicating that the criteria have been met for a Manic Episode, the clinician is instructed to make a rough estimate about the total number of episodes in the patient's lifetime. This entails asking the patient to report how many separate times he or she has had a Manic Episode—it does not mean that the clinician has to inquire about each symptom for each episode.

Skip Instruction. If a Manic Episode has been present, the clinician is instructed to skip the evaluation of a Hypomanic Episode and Dysthymic Disorder and to continue with the assessment of psychotic symptoms (B1). This is because neither Dysthymic Disorder nor Bipolar II Disorder (of which Hypomanic Episode is a critical element) can be diagnosed if there has been a history of Manic Episodes.

Ratings for Hypomanic Episode (items A30–A44)

Criterion A (item A30). Remember that the only way to get here in the SCID is to have a "+" rating on Manic Episode item A16 (i.e., a period of euphoric or irritable mood) that falls short of the required duration of at least 1 week (i.e., a "−" rating on item A17). Therefore, in most cases the clinician needs only to ensure that the duration of the elevated or irritable mood is at least 4 days. Note that the second half of this criterion emphasizes that to rate a mood as "hypomanic," it must be a mood state that is clearly different from the patient's typical euthymic mood. This consideration can be problematic in patients with chronic depression who may experience a return to euthymia as if it were a euphoric mood.

Criterion B (items A31–A38). By definition, a Hypomanic Episode is severe enough to be distinguishable from "normal" good moods (see criteria C and D) but not so severe that it causes marked functional impairment (see criterion E). As can be seen with this criterion, the description of the specific hypomanic symptoms is identical in wording to that in the definition of a Manic Episode and is differentiated solely based on severity.

Criterion C (item A39). To rate this criterion "+," the clinician must ensure that the mood change and other symptoms result in a clear-cut change in functioning (e.g., increased productivity at work) that is not typical of the patient's functioning when not in an episode.

Criterion D (item A40). To further ensure that the mood change is significant, this criterion requires that the change in functioning be observable by others—a subjective sense of elevated mood that is not corroborated by others is not sufficient. In lieu of information from informants, examples of situations in which others commented about the patient's change in behavior are acceptable.

Criterion E (item A41). This criterion is the opposite of criterion C in Manic Episode and requires the absence of significant functional impairment caused by the hypomanic behavior. If significant functional impairment is reported, the clinician should reconsider whether the duration of symptoms is at least a week. If so, the clinician should return to item A26 on page 10 (in the Administration Booklet) and diagnose a Manic Episode. Otherwise, a diagnosis of Bipolar Disorder NOS (in Module D) may be appropriate.

Criterion F (item A42). This criterion instructs the clinician to consider and rule out a general medical condition or a substance as an etiological factor. See pages 10–12 (in the User's Guide) for a general discussion of how to apply this criterion and pages 24–27 (in the User's Guide) for a discussion of the criteria for Mood Disorder Due to a General Medical Condition and Substance-Induced Mood Disorder.

Number of Episodes (item A44). After making a rating of "+" on item A43, indicating that the criteria have been met for a Hypomanic Episode, the clinician is instructed to make a rough estimate about the total number of episodes in the patient's lifetime. This entails asking the patient to report how many separate times he or she has had a Hypomanic Episode—it does not mean that the clinician has to inquire about each symptom for each episode.

Ratings for Dysthymic Disorder (items A45–A60)

In the SCID-CV (unlike in DSM-IV) the diagnosis of Dysthymic Disorder is made only if it is current (i.e., criteria met for at least the past 2 years) because of the difficulty in making a reliable retrospective assessment. In the absence of any current or prior Major Depressive Episodes, the assessment of Dysthymic Disorder is straightforward (i.e., Has there been depressed mood, plus additional depressive symptoms, for more days than not, for the past 2 years?). However, when there is a current or past Major Depressive Episode, making an additional diagnosis of Dysthymic Disorder is more complicated because it is important to distinguish between Dysthymic Disorder with superimposed Major Depressive Disorder (so-called "double depression") and partially remitted Major Depressive Disorder. This differential diagnosis depends on whether the 2-year period of chronic mild depression preceded the onset of the Major Depressive Episode (in which case both diagnoses would be appropriate) or the chronic depressed mood came only after the Major Depressive Episodes (in which case only a diagnosis of Major Depressive Disorder In Partial Remission would apply). Figures 1–5 (page 23) graphically illustrate this differential. Figure 1 shows recurrent Major Depressive Disorder (with full interepisode recovery), and Figure 2 depicts Dysthymic Disorder (without any superimposed Major Depressive Episodes). Figure 3 illustrates Major Depressive Disorder in Partial Remission in which the Major Depressive Episode tapers off into a chronically depressed but less severe mood disturbance. The bottom two drawings illustrate two cases in which it is appropriate to diagnose both Major Depressive Disorder and Dysthymic Disorder. The first (Figure 4) shows a 2-year-plus period of Dysthymic Disorder with a Major Depressive Episode superimposed later in the course. Figure 5 shows a 2-year-plus period of Dysthymic Disorder following a Major Depressive Episode but, in contrast with Figure 3 (which shows Major Depressive Disorder in Partial Remission), there is a 2-month-plus period of remission between the Major Depressive Episode and the onset of the Dysthymic Disorder.

It is not always easy to distinguish a pattern of "double depression" from frequently recurring depressive episodes separated by periods of partial remission, and for many clinical settings this may be an unnecessary distinction. If a clinician is interested only in differentiating chronic depression from recurrent, remitting depression, or in differentiating any depression from no depression, attempts to assess for "double depression" may not justify the time and effort required. In such cases, the clinician may wish to skip the evaluation of Dysthymic Disorder and continue with the assessment of psychotic symptoms on page 25 of the Administration Booklet.

Differential Diagnosis of Major Depressive Disorder and Dysthymic Disorder

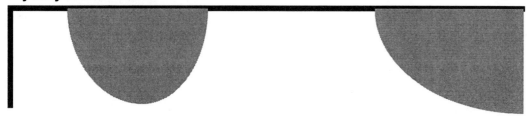

Figure 1.   Major Depressive Disorder, Recurrent

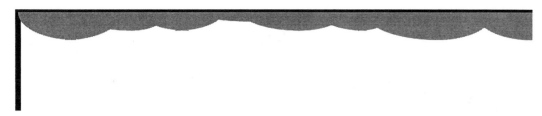

Figure 2.   Dysthymic Disorder

Figure 3.   Major Depressive Disorder in Partial Remission

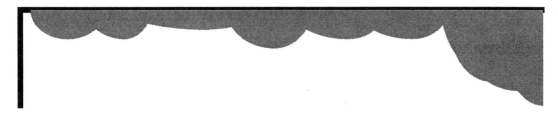

Figure 4.   Major Depressive Disorder superimposed on Dysthymic Disorder ("double depression")

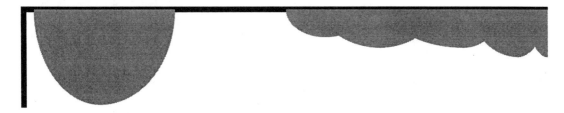

Figure 5.   Dysthymic Disorder; Past Major Depressive Disorder

Criterion A (item A45). The depressed mood characteristic of Dysthymic Disorder need only be present for 50% (or more) of the time. As discussed earlier, in cases in which there have been Major Depressive Episodes in the past 2 years, this question would need to be rephrased so that the clinician is focusing on a 2-year period of depressed mood before the onset of the Major Depressive Episodes. In such situations, it is often helpful for the clinician to draw a figure (such as those in Figures 1–5), indicating the longitudinal course of the depression, for corroboration of the pattern by the patient.

Criterion B (items A46–A52). Items A46, A47, A48, and A50 are identical to the corresponding items for Major Depressive Episode, except that they need not occur nearly every day for at least 2 weeks. All of the symptoms may be intermittent, but must be present more than half of the days in the 2-year period under consideration. Item A49 is set at a lower threshold than the corresponding item in Major Depressive Episode (item A7), in that it requires only low self-esteem, and not a feeling of worthlessness or inappropriate guilt.

Criterion C (item A53). To ensure the chronic nature of Dysthymic Disorder and to differentiate Dysthymic Disorder from recurrent minor depression, the clinician must make sure that the patient never had any significant depression-free periods (i.e., more than 2 months).

Criterion D (item A55). As discussed earlier, whether a chronic depressed mood represents Dysthymic Disorder or Major Depressive Disorder in Partial Remission depends on the severity of the symptoms and the initial onset of the depression. If the disorder begins with a 2-year period of depression that is less severe than a Major Depressive Episode, the diagnosis of Dysthymic Disorder is appropriate. If no such 2-year period can be documented, the depression is better accounted for by a diagnosis of Major Depressive Disorder in Partial Remission with a prolonged depressive prodrome.

Criterion E (item A56). Dysthymic Disorder is "unipolar," i.e., there can never have been any Manic, Mixed, or Hypomanic Episodes.

Criterion F (item A57). Chronic low-level depression is a common associated feature of chronic Schizophrenia and other psychotic disorders. For this reason, Dysthymic Disorder cannot be diagnosed if it occurs ONLY during the course of a psychotic disorder. In most cases, the clinician will know by this point in the SCID-CV whether the patient suffers from a chronic psychotic disorder (even if he or she does not know which specific disorder to diagnose).

Criterion G (item A58). This criterion instructs the clinician to consider and rule out a general medical condition or a substance as an etiological factor. See page 10–12 (in the User's Guide) for a general discussion of how to apply this criterion, and pages 24–27 (in the User's Guide) for a discussion of the criteria for Mood Disorder Due to a General Medical Condition and Substance-Induced Mood Disorder.

Criterion H (item A59). Although clinicians commonly consider Dysthymic Disorder to be a "mild" condition, the impairment caused by long-standing depression can be quite significant.

Skip-Out Instruction. At the conclusion of the evaluation of Dysthymic Disorder, the clinician is instructed to skip to page 25 (in the Administration Booklet) to start the evaluation of psychotic symptoms. The remaining sections of this module (Mood Disorder Due to a General Medical Condition and Substance-Induced Mood Disorder) are evaluated ONLY if there is evidence during the assessment of Major Depressive Episode, Manic Episode, Hypomanic Episode, or Dysthymic Disorder that a general medical condition or substance may have been etiological.

Ratings for Mood Disorder Due to a General Medical Condition/Substance-Induced Mood Disorder (Secondary Mood Disorder) (items A61–A69)

This section of the SCID-CV is consulted only when evaluating the "organic rule out" criterion, which is included in the criteria sets for Major Depressive Episode, Manic Episode, Hypomanic Episode, Dysthymic Disorder, Bipolar Disorder NOS, and Depressive Disorder NOS. The SCID-CV rule is that if there is any indication that a drug of abuse, medication, or general medical condition may be responsible for the mood disturbance through a direct physiological mechanism, the clinician should go to this section to make a more definitive judgment. This section starts with a skip instruction that directs the clinician to consider Mood Disorder Due to a General Medical Condition if a general medical condition is suspected to be causally involved and/or to Substance-Induced Mood Disorder if a substance may be responsible.

Due to a General Medical Condition (items A61–A64). When a general medical condition and mood disturbance co-occur, four relationships are possible: 1) the mood disturbance may be caused by the direct physiological effects of the general medical condition on the central nervous system (e.g., brain tumor or hypothyroidism causing depression); 2) the mood disturbance may be a psychological reaction to having the general medical condition (e.g., depression in response to physical disability caused by a stroke); 3) the mood disturbance may be caused by the direct physiological effects of a medication used to treat the general medical condition; and 4) the two may be coincidental. The clinician's task here is to distinguish the first relationship (which would lead to a diagnosis of Mood Disorder Due to a General Medical Condition) from the other three.

Criterion A (item A61). This criterion is included for completeness and is essentially automatically coded "+" (i.e., you would be here only if there were depressed, elevated, or irritable mood that you suspect is due to a general medical condition).

Criterion B/C (item A62). In the SCID-CV, these two DSM-IV criteria have been combined into a single item because they are essentially flip sides of the same concept. Rating this criterion entails the often difficult (and sometimes impossible to make) judgment that the general medical condition is etiologically responsible for the mood disturbance. Please note that whereas depression is commonly comorbid with a general medical condition, Mood Disorder Due to a General Medical Condition is relatively rare. Therefore, when in doubt, the clinician's default position should be to assume that the medical condition is NOT etiological (i.e., the mood disorder is primary). Although DSM-IV does not provide specific criteria for making this determination, the SCID-CV

includes four guidelines derived from the DSM-IV text that may be helpful:

1. *Is it reasonably well established in the medical literature that mood disturbance may be caused by the general medical condition?* For example, hypothyroidism is a well documented cause of depression, whereas gastric ulcer is not.

2. *Is there a close temporal relationship between the course of the mood symptoms and the course of the general medical condition?* Do the mood symptoms start following the onset of the general medical condition, get better or worse with the waxing and waning of the general medical condition, and remit when the general medical condition is resolved? The questions provided in the left-hand column of the SCID-CV address these relationships. When all of these relationships can be demonstrated, one can make a fairly compelling case that there is a causal connection between the mood symptoms and the general medical condition. It is important to note that demonstration of a close temporal relationship does not necessarily imply that the causality is on a physiological level—a psychological reaction would likely have a close temporal relationship as well. Furthermore, the lack of a temporal relationship does not necessarily rule out causality. In some instances, mood symptoms may be the first harbinger of the general medical condition and may precede by months or years any physical manifestations (e.g., brain tumor). Conversely, mood symptoms may be a relatively late manifestation, occurring months or years following the onset of the general medical condition.

3. *Are the mood symptoms characterized by atypical presenting features (e.g., late age at onset)?* For example, severe weight loss in the face of a relatively mild depression, or the first onset of mania in an elderly patient, increases the likelihood that a general medical condition is responsible. It should be realized, however, that atypicality is not necessarily compelling evidence because by their nature, psychiatric presentations are heterogeneous within a particular diagnosis.

4. *Are there no reasonable alternative explanations?* Has the patient had prior episodes of mood disturbance not due to a general medical condition? Is the patient abusing substances

that can cause mood disturbance or taking a medication that might cause a mood disturbance? Does the patient have a strong family history of mood disorders?

Because these guidelines are potentially fallible, they should all be considered and, ultimately, the final decision rests on clinical judgment. Because of the inherent difficulty in making this judgment, we recommend that clinicians working in a particular setting establish a policy with respect to the threshold of evidence required to justify a decision that the general medical condition is etiological. As discussed earlier, Mood Disorder Due to a General Medical Condition is relatively rare so that it probably makes sense to maintain a high threshold (i.e., when in doubt, do not diagnose Mood Disorder Due to a General Medical Condition). However, in settings in which it is particularly important to screen out possible etiological general medical conditions, it may make sense to establish a very low threshold (i.e., any possible associated general medical condition would be considered etiological and would trigger a medical consultation).

Substance-Induced (items A65–A69). This section begins with a skip-out instruction that tells you to "return to the episode being evaluated" if there is no temporal association between the mood symptoms and a substance, an instruction that repeats itself throughout pages 22–23 of the Administration Booklet. Recall that the only way to arrive at the evaluation of the Substance-Induced items is to have jumped here from an item located earlier in the SCID. For example, in the course of evaluating item A12 for a Major Depressive Episode (i.e., the mood is not due to the direct physiological effects of a substance), the clinician is instructed to jump here if there is evidence that substance use may have played an etiological role. Therefore, you must return to the section of the SCID-CV that sent you here, after completing the ratings of the Substance-Induced criteria.

When substance use and mood symptoms co-occur, there are three possibilities as to the nature of their relationship: 1) the mood symptoms may be a direct physiological consequence of the substance use (e.g., Cocaine-Induced Mood Disorder, With Depressive Features, With Onset During Withdrawal); 2) the substance use may be a feature of the mood disorder (e.g., cocaine use to self-medicate an underlying depressive disor-

der); and 3) the two may be coincidental. The ratings for Substance-Induced Mood Disorder involve differentiating the first causal connection from the other two. It should be recalled that in DSM-IV, the term "substance use" includes the use of prescribed medication, as well as somatic therapies such as electroconvulsive treatment and phototherapy.

Criterion A (item A65). This criterion is included for completeness and is essentially automatically coded "+" (i.e., you would be here only if there is depressed, elevated, or irritable mood that you suspect is due to a substance).

Criterion B (item A66). This criterion establishes a temporal relationship between substance use and the development of the mood symptoms. Part (1) of this criterion applies to drugs of abuse whereas Part (2) applies to medication use. For drugs of abuse, this criterion establishes that the mood symptoms occur in the context of the full intoxication or withdrawal syndrome associated with that substance, thereby implying that enough of the substance was used to have caused intoxication or withdrawal.

Criterion C (item A67). Given that there is a temporal relationship between the onset of the mood symptoms and substance use (as per criterion B), this criterion asks you to consider whether there is any non-substance-related explanation that better accounts for the mood symptoms. If not, you can assume that there is an etiological connection between the mood symptoms and the substance use. Four suggested guidelines are presented:

1. *Does the substance use clearly follow the onset of the mood symptoms?* If so, the mood clearly cannot be caused by the substance use and instead the "self-medication" model would seem to apply.

2. *Do the mood symptoms persist, even after a substantial period of abstinence (e.g., a month)?* If the mood symptoms are caused by the substance use, then one would expect that they would remit after the acute effects of intoxication and withdrawal subside. If the mood symptoms continue to persist long after the substance use ends, it suggests instead that the mood symptoms represent a primary mood disorder (or perhaps a Mood Disorder due to a

General Medical Condition). Note that the 1-month period is only a loose guideline. The actual amount of time of abstinence that would be required before concluding that the mood symptoms are primary depends on many factors, such as the particular substance used and dosage.

3. *Are the mood symptoms much more severe than one would expect given the nature and amount of the substance used?* If so, then it would not make sense to attribute the mood symptoms to the substance (e.g., severe depression following a small amount of cocaine use suggests Major Depressive Disorder rather than Cocaine-Induced Mood Disorder).

4. *Is there any other evidence that is more supportive of a primary Mood Disorder or a Mood Disorder Due to a General Medical Condition?* The interviewer should consider factors such as a strong family history of primary Mood Disorder, prior episodes of Mood Disorder that were not related to substance use, and evidence for an etiological general medical condition.

Note that these are only examples of scenarios that suggest a non-substance-related explanation and do not conclusively rule out a substance-induced disorder. Clinical judgment must be applied.

9.4 Module B. Psychotic and Associated Symptoms

Module B is for rating the lifetime occurrence of psychotic and other symptoms (e.g., delusions, hallucinations, disorganized speech and behavior, and negative symptoms) included in the criteria sets for the Psychotic Disorders. Ratings for the specific criteria are contained in Module C (i.e., ratings for Schizophrenia, Schizophreniform, Schizoaffective, and Brief Psychotic Disorders, Psychotic Disorder Due to a General Medical Condition, and Substance-Induced Psychotic Disorder) and Module D (i.e., ratings for Bipolar I Disorder or Bipolar II Disorder With Psychotic Features and Major Depressive Disorder With Psychotic Features). Because the clinician is assessing lifetime psychotic symptoms, it is necessary to date occurrences of specific symptoms. If a patient is too psychotic or disorganized to complete a SCID-CV interview, the evidence for psy-

chotic symptoms will come from medical records. In such situations, the SCID-CV can be used as a place to document symptoms and to apply the diagnostic algorithms in the C module rather than as a structured interview.

Interviewing for Psychotic Symptoms. In most patients with a Psychotic Disorder, the presence of a psychotic symptom has been established earlier in the interview (usually in the Overview). In such instances, the B module may serve more as a checklist for rating psychotic symptoms rather than an interview guide. In fact, this is the one part of the SCID-CV where the rule requiring the interviewer to paraphrase a question into a confirmatory question if the answer is already known does not apply. For example, if the clinician has already established during the Overview that the patient believes that he is God, there is no need to say "you've told me that you are especially important in some way or that you have the power to do things that other people couldn't do." It is still important to ask all patients (even those who have reported some psychotic symptoms) those questions assessing psychotic symptoms that have not yet been reported because they are useful both as a general screen for psychotic symptoms and to determine the full range of psychotic symptoms in patients with a psychotic disorder.

Rating Delusions (items B1–B5). A *delusion* is a false personal belief based on incorrect inference about external reality that is firmly sustained despite what others believe and despite what constitutes incontrovertible and obvious proof or evidence to the contrary. The belief is not one ordinarily accepted by other members of the patient's culture or subculture (e.g., the belief in some cultures that one can communicate with a dead person). When the clinician is unfamiliar with the beliefs characteristic of the patient's cultural or religious background, consultation with someone who is familiar with the patient's culture may be required to avoid the overdiagnosis of delusions.

A delusion involves impairment in the ability to make logical inferences—the way conclusions are drawn from observation of the person's environment or self (e.g., being convinced that phone hang-ups indicate that the person is being spied on). In rating each type of delusion, the clinician must differentiate a delusion (which would warrant a rating of "+") from a strongly held "overvalued" idea (which would warrant a rating of "–"). For example, a patient who frequently gets the feeling that people are talking about him when he walks down the street but knows that it might be his imagination would be considered to have an overvalued idea. In contrast, a patient who is completely convinced that strangers are talking about him would have a delusion of reference.

In deciding whether a belief is false and fixed enough to be considered a delusion, the clinician must first determine that a serious error in inference and reality testing has occurred and then determine the strength of the conviction. It may be helpful to ask the patient to talk at length about his conviction because it is often only in the specific details that the errors of inference become apparent. In evaluating the strength of the delusional conviction, the clinician should present alternative explanations (e.g., is it possible that the phone hang-ups are a result of people dialing a wrong number?). A delusional patient may acknowledge the possibility of these explanations but will still hold firm to his or her own belief. Some patients with a long-standing history of psychotic disorder have developed insight into the "psychotic" nature of their delusions. Such a symptom would still be considered psychotic if, at some earlier point, the symptom was experienced as real. For example, a patient may report that his chronic conviction that people at work are plotting against him is a result of his long-standing Schizophrenia. This would be coded as a delusion either if the patient reports that initially he was convinced the plot was real or if there is such evidence from prior records (e.g., an admission note documenting that he acted on his belief).

The next set of ratings documents the type of delusion based on content. Note that for a particular delusion, more than one rating may apply. For example, a patient who believes that the FBI is after him because he can control other people's minds would have both persecutory and grandiose types of delusions coded "+."

Delusion of Reference (item B1). "Yes" answers to this question are relatively common and usually do not indicate a delusion of reference. The clinician should therefore follow up by asking for specific examples that establish the psychotic nature of the belief. Most people have at sometime thought that other people were talking about them, particularly if they have some obvious physical abnormality or act in a conspicuous way.

It is therefore important to differentiate realistic perceptions, social anxiety, or transient suspiciousness from a fixed false belief. A homeless man who dresses in rags and has no place to take a shower may realistically believe that people are moving away from him on the subway, but if he believes that current headlines are a cryptic reference to his personal life, the clinician should rate this item as "+."

Persecutory Delusion (item B2). The clinician should carefully differentiate an exaggerated, but possibly valid, perception of persecution (e.g., by a boss, a teacher, an ex-spouse, a drug dealer) from a real persecutory delusion. There may be cases in which it is impossible to know whether the persecution is real or delusional. These should be coded "?."

Grandiose Delusion (item B3). It is sometimes hard to tell where an inflated perception of one's talents ends and a grandiose delusion begins. A taxi driver who believes she will write a best-selling novel may be mistaken but not necessarily delusional. If, however, that person tells the interviewer that Steven Spielberg has been calling and begging for the movie rights to her novel, she has probably stepped over the line into delusion. Questioning the patient about her evidence for the belief is a good way to clarify the issue.

Somatic Delusion (item B4). In assessing this symptom, it is necessary to consider the patient's understanding of anatomy and physiology. An uneducated person may have a primitive explanation of symptoms, for example, that stomach pains are caused by a grasshopper hopping around inside her. The patient's willingness to seriously entertain an alternative explanation indicates that the belief is not a delusion. Another example where a "yes" answer does not indicate a somatic delusion would be a patient with physical symptoms who doubts an internist's reassurance that she has no medical illness. If the patient is able to entertain the possibility that her beliefs are exaggerated, then the diagnosis is more likely Hypochondriasis. A patient who dismisses such reassurances out of hand is more likely to have a somatic delusion.

Other Delusions (item B5). Other types of delusions that do not easily fit into one of the specified types are coded here (e.g., delusional jealousy).

Auditory Hallucinations (item B6). Auditory hallucinations typically involve hearing voices, although some patients report hearing music or noises. This item should be coded "+" only if the hallucinations are judged to be clinically significant (i.e., recurrent or persistent). Hearing one's name being called and finding no one there is an example of a hallucination that is not clinically significant. True auditory hallucinations should be distinguished from delusions of reference, in which the patient hears actual voices (on the street, on the ward, etc.) and interprets them self-referentially. Evidence that they are, in fact, hallucinations might be that the patient hears voices even when the patient is alone.

Visual and Other Hallucinations (items B7–B9). Hallucinations in modalities other than auditory are especially likely to have a substance or general medical etiology. The clinician should take this into account in Module C when considering whether a psychotic presentation is due to the direct physiological effects of a substance or general medical condition (e.g., when rating item C6 in Schizophrenia). A hallucination (the experience of sensory perception without stimulation of the relevant sensory organ) should be distinguished from an illusion, which is a misperception of an actual stimulus (e.g., misinterpreting a shadow as the figure of a person) and would warrant a rating of "–."

Catatonic Behaviors (item B10). This item is almost always coded based on historical information from other informants or after a review of prior records because patients with current catatonia are unable to provide such information. Catatonia may involve motoric immobility, excessive motor activity, extreme negativism, mutism, perculiarities of voluntary movement, echolalia, or echopraxia. Motoric immobility may be manifested by catalepsy (waxy flexibility) or stupor. The excessive motor activity characteristic of catatonic agitation is apparently purposeless and is not influenced by external stimuli. There may be extreme negativism that is manifested by the maintenance of a rigid posture against attempts to be moved or resistance to all instructions. Peculiarities of voluntary movement are manifested by the assumption of inappropriate or bizarre postures or by prominent grimacing. Echolalia is the pathological, parrot-like, and apparently senseless repetition of a word or phrase just spoken by another person. Echopraxia is the repetitive imitation of

the movements of another person. Additional features include stereotypies, mannerisms, and automatic obedience or mimicry. Note that some of these symptoms, such as catatonic excitement and catatonic immobility, differ only in degree from mood symptoms such as agitation and retardation. For example, slowing down of movements that causes a patient to spend 2 hours getting dressed would be evidence for psychomotor retardation, whereas complete immobility for several hours would be considered catatonia.

Grossly Disorganized Behavior (item B11). Two judgments are required here—that the behavior is "disorganized" and that it is severely so ("grossly"). Disorganized behavior does not have any apparent goal. Examples of disorganized behavior include wandering around aimlessly and unpredictably shouting at passersby. It is important to exclude behavior that may appear disorganized or bizarre but in fact has a goal (e.g., collecting worthless items from trash dumpsters in response to a delusion that they would provide protection against radiation). To justify a rating of "+," the disorganized behavior must be severely impairing and obvious even to the most casual observer.

Grossly Inappropriate Affect (item B12). As with the previous item, the inappropriateness of the display of affect must be particularly extreme to justify a rating of "+" (e.g., a patient who laughs while talking about his father's unexpected death in a car accident 2 years ago).

Disorganized Speech (item B13). This item is usually assessed by history and almost always requires another informant. If the patient's speech is disorganized enough to warrant a rating of "+," it may be impossible to administer the SCID-CV.

The assessment of this criterion requires a subjective judgment by the clinician as to the "understandability" of the patient's speech. The most common error is to have too low a threshold for disorganization, leading to an overdiagnosis of Schizophrenia. It is unwise to assume that every subtle illogical shift from one topic to another necessarily has pathological significance. Latitude should be given to account for variations in style, particularly in the stressful situation of a psychiatric interview. Only speech that is severely disorganized and very difficult to interpret should be considered for a rating of "+." A final caution is that the clinician's unfamiliarity with the patient's dialect or accent or the patient's lack of proficiency in the clinician's language should not be misdiagnosed as disorganized speech.

Negative Symptoms (item B14). This item is restricted to the three negative symptoms (affective flattening, alogia, avolition) that have been included in the definition of Schizophrenia. *Affective flattening* is characterized by the patient's face appearing immobile and unresponsive, with poor eye contact and reduced body language. Although a person with affective flattening may smile and seem happy occasionally, the range of emotional expressiveness is clearly diminished most of the time. It may be useful to observe the patient interacting with peers to determine whether affective flattening is sufficiently persistent to meet the criterion. *Alogia* (poverty of speech) is manifested by brief, laconic, and empty replies. The patient with alogia appears to have a diminution of thoughts that is reflected in decreased fluency and productivity of speech. This must be differentiated from an unwillingness to speak, a clinical judgment that may require observation over time and in a variety of situations. *Avolition* is characterized by an inability to initiate and persist in goal-directed activities. The patient may sit for long periods of time and show little interest in participating in work or social activities. Avolition can be assessed historically by asking the patient questions about his or her daily activities.

The main problem with the assessment of negative symptoms is too low a threshold for judging the symptom present. Like disorganized speech and grossly disorganized behavior, there is a continuum of severity for each of the negative symptoms and only the most severe, pervasive, persistent, and impairing forms should warrant a rating of "+" for this item. For example, the range of affective expression varies widely in the population and among different cultural groups. Many people are laconic without having negative symptoms. The lack of goal direction meant to be conveyed by the term "avolition" is at the extreme end of a spectrum and should not be confused with lesser and more common difficulties in getting started.

Furthermore, it is important to ensure that other explanations for the behavior be considered and ruled out before rating this item a "+." The most common confusion in this regard is probably because the very medications used to treat psy-

chotic disorders can produce side effects that appear to be negative symptoms. For example, many patients on antipsychotic medication experience loss of facial expressiveness, reduced speech and movements, dysphoria, and loss of energy. It may be useful to inquire whether negative symptoms were present before the onset of the neuroleptic treatment, and a reduction or change in medication or the addition of an anticholinergic agent may sometimes be informative. It can also be difficult to distinguish between negative symptoms (affective flattening, alogia, and avolition) and depressive symptoms (constricted affect, psychomotor retardation, indecisiveness, loss of energy, and loss of pleasure) that frequently accompany psychotic disorders. Finally, negative symptoms must be differentiated from behaviors that are secondary to positive symptoms. For example, a patient experiencing a command hallucination to remain perfectly silent would not also be considered to have the negative symptom alogia. Similarly, a patient who is unable to maintain a job because of persecutory delusions would not also be considered as having avolition.

9.5 Module C. Psychotic Disorders

Module C allows the clinician to make a differential diagnosis of Psychotic Disorders based on information obtained in the A and B modules. The Psychotic Disorders module is skipped if there has never been a psychotic symptom or if the psychotic symptoms occur only during mood episodes.

This module is different from Modules A and B in several ways. The primary goal in Modules A and B is to collect specific information from the patient (and/or other informants) about the clinical presentation to determine whether individual criteria are met, whereas the goal in Module C is to determine which psychotic disorder best accounts for the particular symptomatic presentation. Proceeding through Module C is equivalent to moving down the DSM-IV decision tree for psychotic symptoms (pages 694–695). The main focus of the clinician's efforts is on the consideration of whether the criterion in the box is present or absent. A rating of "yes" is made if the criterion is met and a rating of "no" applies if the criterion is not met. If the clinician is unable to decide whether or not the criterion has been met because of missing information (e.g., the patient is a poor historian, old charts are unavailable, etc.), the clinician has the option of skipping to item C34 and making a diagnosis of Psychotic Disorder Not Otherwise Specified. Because many of the items are complicated and involve double negatives, notes are provided below many of the criterion items as a quick guide to what the ratings mean. It is suggested that you review the notes before making a final rating to confirm that you have correctly interpreted the criterion item.

For most items in Module C, there is no need to ask a question, although for some items, one or two additional clarification questions are provided in a dashed box. In many cases the last thing said to the patient (until Module E) is the phrase "Let me stop for a minute while I make a few notes" after item B9 on page 27 (in the Administration Booklet). The clinician then proceeds to rate the criteria and flip through pages while the patient observes. Alternatively, the clinician might ask the patient to take a 10-minute break while he or she completes Modules C and D, and then bring the patient back for any additional questions. In any case, Modules C and D must be completed before the patient is "released" from the interview. We recommend that the clinician become proficient in using this section so it can be done quickly so that patient is not waiting too long while each word in Module C is pondered. The case examples in the Appendix are particularly helpful for practicing how to use Module C.

Note that there are two situations in which the clinician may have to go *back* to the A module to recode items: 1) if the diagnosis of Dysthymic Disorder was made in the A module and then a psychotic disorder diagnosis is made in the C module, item A57 in Dysthymic Disorder (i.e., "does not occur exclusively during the course of a chronic Psychotic Disorder") may have to be recoded; OR 2) because of the difficulty in distinguishing the negative symptoms of Schizophrenia from symptoms of depression, a Major Depressive Episode that has been previously diagnosed in the A module might have to be recoded if a diagnosis of Schizophrenia is made in the C module. In these cases, the clinician should return to the A module and recode any equivocal items as "–" if they are determined to be negative symptoms of Schizophrenia.

Recurrent Psychotic Episodes. Some psychotic disorders tend to be chronic (i.e., Schizophrenia, Delusional Disorder), whereas others tend to be more episodic (Mood Disorder With Psychotic

Features, Schizoaffective Disorder). Although most patients with recurrent psychotic episodes have recurrences that are characterized by similar symptom presentations, there are rare cases in which the presentation markedly changes from episode to episode. For example, one episode may meet criteria for Bipolar Disorder with Psychotic Features (e.g., delusions confined to a Manic Episode), while another episode meets the criteria for Schizoaffective Disorder (delusions persist for 2 weeks after the Manic Episode has resolved). In such circumstances, we recommend that only the current (or most recent) episode be diagnosed.

Rule Out Psychotic Mood Disorder (item C1)

The hallmark of a Mood Disorder With Psychotic Features is that psychotic symptoms occur only during Mood Episodes. This initial criterion (which is not actually part of the criteria set for any DSM-IV disorder) has been included in the SCID-CV to allow the clinician to skip the evaluation of nonmood psychotic disorders.

Ratings for Schizophrenia (items C2–C12)

Criterion A (item C2). This criterion defines the "active phase" of Schizophrenia, which is required at some point during the patient's lifetime for a diagnosis of Schizophrenia to be warranted. Note that in some cases the active phase symptoms may have been present many years before the interview. This criterion requires that there be an active phase lasting at least 1 month, or less if successfully treated. This last phrase acknowledges that clinical judgment is required when applying the duration criterion. In a patient who has been promptly and aggressively treated with antipsychotic medication and the other aspects of the illness are unequivocally present, it does not make sense to require a full month's duration.

Criterion D (item C3). For presentations characterized by a mixture of mood and psychotic symptoms that meet criterion A for Schizophrenia, the differential diagnosis includes Schizophrenia, Schizoaffective Disorder, and Mood Disorder With Psychotic Features. As discussed earlier, the clinician has already been instructed to skip Module C if the diagnosis is Mood Disorder With Psychotic Features. This criterion delineates the admittedly inexact boundary between Schizophrenia and Schizoaffective Disorder. A "yes" rating indicates that the clinician has ruled out Schizoaffective Disorder and the SCID-CV then continues with item C4 for Schizophrenia. A "no" rating indicates that a diagnosis of Schizoaffective Disorder is likely and that the interview should continue with item C16 on page 35 (in the Administration Booklet). **Note:** This criterion is presented in a different order than in DSM-IV to maximize diagnostic efficiency.

The two essential aspects of the boundary between Schizophrenia and Schizoaffective Disorder are represented by the two parts of the criterion. The first part indicates the requirement in Schizoaffective Disorder that mood episodes occur concurrently with the active phase symptoms of Schizophrenia (corresponding to criterion A in Schizoaffective Disorder). If this is not the case, then Schizoaffective Disorder is ruled out on this point alone and the interview can continue with Schizophrenia criterion C. Note that this criterion is a double negative—FOLLOW THE INSTRUCTIONS IN THE NOTE TO PREVENT A WRONG TURN! If there is an overlap between the mood episodes and psychotic symptoms (suggesting Schizoaffective Disorder), the clinician must then evaluate the second half of the criterion to determine the duration of the mood symptoms compared with the total disturbance. Schizophrenia is the diagnosis if the mood component of the disturbance has been BRIEF relative to the total duration of the disturbance; Schizoaffective Disorder is more likely if the mood symptoms constitute a SIGNIFICANT aspect of the total duration. (AGAIN—the second half of this criterion is also awkward to use—READ THE NOTE FOR GUIDANCE.)

Unfortunately, to the distress of most SCIDers, neither DSM-IV nor this User's Guide can precisely define "brief" versus "significant." It is a clinical judgment that is certainly one of the sources of unreliability in this diagnosis.

Even if DSM-IV had a precise definition of "brief," it would still be a difficult criterion to assess reliably because patients (and patient charts) generally cannot tell you about the relative persistence of mood episodes versus psychotic symptoms. At one end of the spectrum is the 40-year-old who was depressed and suicidal for a few months when he had his first psychotic episode at age 20 but has gone on to a 20-year career of waxing and waning psychotic symptoms, without additional mood episodes. In this situa-

tion, the mood episode was clearly "brief" relative to the duration of the psychotic symptoms, so Schizoaffective Disorder was ruled out (i.e., the coding on item C3 was "yes") and the clinician went on to assess the other criteria for Schizophrenia. At the other end of the spectrum is someone who has become severely depressed for months every time there has been an exacerbation of his psychotic symptoms. The total duration of his mood episodes is clearly not brief relative to the total duration of the disorder, so the clinician codes "no" and goes on to assess for Schizoaffective Disorder. The problem is that in the real world, most patients fall somewhere in the middle of this spectrum, and there is no precise cut point. One possible guideline that has been used defines brief as 10% of the time or less. In those cases where the clinician is unable to make a rating of either "yes" or "no" because of missing information, the clinician has the option of jumping to item C39 and making a diagnosis of Psychotic Disorder Not Otherwise Specified. Depressive Disorder Not Otherwise Specified (item D19) or Bipolar Disorder Not Otherwise Specified (item D12) can also be diagnosed to indicate the significant mood symptomatology.

Criterion C (item C4). The 6-month duration criterion, which differentiates between Schizophrenia and Schizophreniform Disorder, is generally an issue only in first-break patients. Note that the 6-month duration includes any combination of active, prodromal, and residual symptoms.

DSM-III and DSM-III-R contained lists of specific prodromal and residual symptoms. DSM-IV has replaced these with a simpler definition of residual and prodromal symptoms. A patient is considered to be in the prodromal or residual phase of Schizophrenia if, in the absence of concurrent positive symptoms, there are considerable negative symptoms equivalent to those present during the active phase (see criterion A(5) in item C2). Alternatively, the patient can be considered to be in the prodromal or residual phase if there are milder versions of the symptoms listed in criteria A(1)–A(4) above. For example, before becoming frankly delusional or after recovering from delusions, the patient may have overvalued ideas, ideas of reference, or magical thinking with content similar to what is a delusional conviction in the active phase. Similarly, the patient who experiences hallucinations during the active phase may have unusual perceptual experiences in the prodromal or residual phases (e.g., recurrent illusions, perceptions of auras, sensing a force). Disorganized speech that is incoherent during the active phase may be digressive, vague, or over-elaborate in the prodromal or residual phases. The patient may continue to act in a peculiar fashion but no longer exhibit grossly disorganized behavior.

Criterion B (item C5). Functional impairment resulting from the above symptoms is usually quite evident from the Overview, so this is a question that you will rarely need to ask.

Criterion E (item C6). This criterion instructs the clinician to consider and rule out a general medical condition or a substance as an etiological factor. See pages 10–12 (in the User's Guide) for a general discussion of how to apply this criterion and pages 24–27 (in the User's Guide) for a discussion of the criteria for a Mood Disorder Due to a General Medical Condition and a Substance-Induced Mood Disorder, which also apply to Psychotic Disorder Due to a General Medical Condition and Substance-Induced Psychotic Disorder. Note that the presence of certain psychotic symptoms (e.g., hallucinations in modalities other than auditory) or an atypical course (e.g., first onset of psychotic symptoms after age 60) strongly suggests the possibility of a general medical or substance etiology.

If the patient has had a primary psychotic disorder but also has psychotic symptoms due to a General Medical Condition/Substance, both can be diagnosed by repeating Module C (i.e., one time for the primary psychotic symptoms and a second time for the "organic psychosis"). For this reason, there is an instruction in the box under the "no" arrow to go back to item C2 and start the decision tree again after making a diagnosis of General Medical Condition/Substance-Induced Psychotic Disorder if there is evidence that the patient has also had psychotic symptoms at other times (i.e., when not using substances or suffering from a general medical condition).

Schizophrenia Subtypes (items C8–C12). Once a diagnosis of Schizophrenia is made, the clinician is instructed to determine which subtype is relevant to describe the current clinical state. Note that the diagnostic code for Schizophrenia requires a determination of the particular subtype.

Ratings for Schizophreniform Disorder (items C13–C15)

The SCID-CV resumes at this point if criteria A and D of Schizophrenia are present (i.e., active phase symptoms for at least a month, and Schizoaffective Disorder has been ruled out) but criterion C is not true (i.e., total duration is NOT greater than 6 months). Part of criterion A for Schizophreniform Disorder has already been assessed during the evaluation for Schizophrenia (item C2) so the assessment for Schizophreniform Disorder begins with criterion B.

Criterion B (item C13). It is important to ensure that the symptoms have lasted at least 1 month because it is possible to have jumped to this point in the SCID-CV for a patient with a period of psychotic symptoms that have lasted for less than 1 month (e.g., delusions and hallucinations that remitted after 2 weeks as a result of successful treatment with neuroleptics). For symptoms lasting less than 1 month, a diagnosis of Brief Psychotic Disorder is made.

Criterion A (item C14). This criterion instructs the clinician to consider and rule out a general medical condition or a substance as an etiological factor. See pages 10–12 (of the User's Guide) for a general discussion of how to apply this criterion and pages 24–27 (of the User's Guide) for a discussion of the criteria for a Mood Disorder Due to a General Medical Condition and a Substance-Induced Mood Disorder, which also apply to Psychotic Disorder Due to a General Medical Condition and Substance-Induced Psychotic Disorder.

Ratings for Schizoaffective Disorder (items C16–C20)

The SCID-CV resumes here if criterion A for Schizophrenia has been determined to be present (i.e., active phase symptoms for at least a month) *but* criteria D(1) and D(2) for Schizophrenia are not (i.e., there is a period of overlap between Mood Episodes and psychotic symptoms, AND the total duration of the mood episodes is not brief relative to the total duration of the disturbance).

Criterion A (item C16). Item C3 in Schizophrenia, the rough converse of this criterion (i.e., specifying no overlap between the mood and psychotic symptoms), has already been rated "–" on page 30 of the Administration Booklet. This criterion reflects the fact that Schizoaffective Disorder combines elements of Schizophrenia and Mood Disorder. Although no actual number of days is given explicitly in this criterion, it is implied that the minimum duration of a Major Depressive Episode, Manic Episode, or Mixed Episode applies. Therefore, the minimum duration for the overlap of mood and psychotic symptoms that make up criterion A would be 2 weeks if the patient is depressed or 1 week if manic. In clinical practice, however, the actual durations of overlap are usually much longer, comprising months or even years.

It can be a clinical challenge to sort out the degree to which particular behaviors reflect a mood episode, criterion A of Schizophrenia, medication side effects, or some combination of the three. For example, it is sometimes inherently impossible to distinguish depressive symptoms from negative symptoms or from medication side effects. It is sometimes equally difficult to determine whether to attribute disorganized excited behavior to criterion A of Schizophrenia or to a Manic Episode. Note the requirement in criterion A that the Major Depressive Episode in Schizoaffective Disorder must include depressed mood (and not just decreased interest or pleasure). This is an attempt to sharpen the distinction between the definition of a Major Depressive Episode and criterion A of Schizophrenia because it is impossible to determine whether loss of interest is part of a depressive episode or is better accounted for as avolition or anhedonia of Schizophrenia.

Criterion B (item C17). This criterion distinguishes Schizoaffective Disorder from Mood Disorder With Psychotic Features. In a prototypical psychotic Mood Disorder, the psychotic features are confined to the episodes of the Mood Disorder. In contrast, in an episode of Schizoaffective Disorder, the psychotic symptoms either precede the mood symptoms or persist after the mood symptoms significantly improve. In Schizoaffective Disorder, the delusions and/or hallucinations usually persist in the absence of mood symptoms for much longer than the required 2 weeks.

Criterion C (item C18). This is the reverse of the D(2) criterion for Schizophrenia (item C3). See the discussion of Schizophrenia criterion D (page 31 of the User's Guide) for more details.

Criterion D (item C19). This criterion instructs the clinician to consider and rule out a general medical condition or a substance as an etiological factor for both the mood and psychotic symptoms. See pages 10–12 (of the User's Guide) for a general discussion of how to apply this criterion and pages 24–27 (of the User's Guide) for a discussion of the criteria for a Mood Disorder Due to a General Medical Condition and a Substance-Induced Mood Disorder, which also apply to Psychotic Disorder Due to a General Medical Condition and Substance-Induced Psychotic Disorder.

Ratings for Delusional Disorder (items C21–C26)

The SCID-CV resumes here if criterion A for Schizophrenia is not met, thus ruling out Schizophrenia, Schizophreniform Disorder, and Schizoaffective Disorder.

Criteria A and B (items C21 and C22). Delusional Disorder is defined as at least a month of nonbizarre delusions that occur generally in the absence of other psychotic symptoms. However, according to criterion B, some accompanying psychotic symptoms may be present, so long as they are not prominent enough to meet the requirements of criterion A for Schizophrenia (i.e., "present for a significant portion of time during a 1-month period or less if successfully treated"). An exception is made to allow for chronic olfactory or tactile hallucinations that are thematically related to the delusion (e.g., a patient having the perception of emitting a foul body odor related to the delusion that neighbors are avoiding him).

Criterion C (item C23). In contrast to Schizophrenia, a patient with Delusional Disorder will often appear to have no mental illness as long as the clinician has not tapped into the delusional system.

Criterion D (item C24). Analogous to criterion D in Schizophrenia, this criterion indicates the differential diagnosis for patients with mood episodes and long-standing delusions. If the delusions occur exclusively during Mood Episodes, then the diagnosis is Mood Disorder With Psychotic Features rather than Delusional Disorder, and the clinician is instructed to skip to Module D. In contrast, if the patient has persistent and prominent delusions for many years with only occasional and relatively brief mood episodes, the presentation is consistent with Delusional Disorder and the clinician is instructed to continue to evaluate the remaining criteria. The middle ground, analogous to Schizoaffective Disorder, in which persistent delusions are accompanied by significant mood symptoms, is not covered by any specific category in DSM-IV. Such presentations of persistent delusions accompanied by substantial periods of mood symptoms are diagnosed Psychotic Disorder NOS with an accompanying diagnosis of either Depressive Disorder NOS or Bipolar Disorder NOS to indicate the mood episodes. For more specific instructions, see the discussion for item C3 (criterion D of Schizophrenia) on page 31 of the User's Guide.

Criterion E (item C25). This criterion instructs the clinician to consider and rule out a general medical condition or a substance as an etiological factor for both the mood and psychotic symptoms. See pages 10–12 of the User's Guide for a general discussion of how to apply this criterion and pages 24–27 (of the User's Guide) for a discussion of the criteria for a Mood Disorder Due to a General Medical Condition and a Substance-Induced Mood Disorder, which also apply to Psychotic Disorder Due to a General Medical Condition and Substance-Induced Psychotic Disorder.

Ratings for Brief Psychotic Disorder (items C27–C31)

This is a rare diagnosis that applies to psychotic episodes that last at least 1 day, but less than 1 month, and are not part of a Mood Disorder or any of the more specific Psychotic Disorders described earlier, or involve a general medical condition or substance.

Ratings for Psychotic Disorder Due to a General Medical Condition/Substance-Induced Psychotic Disorder (items C32–C38)

This section of the SCID-CV is consulted only in the course of evaluating the "organic rule out" criterion that is included in the criteria sets for Schizophrenia, Schizophreniform Disorder, Schizoaffective Disorder, Delusional Disorder, and Brief Psychotic Disorder. The SCID-CV rule is that if there is any indication that a drug of abuse, medication, or general medical condition may be responsible for the psychotic symptoms

through a direct physiological mechanism, the clinician should jump to this section to make a more definitive judgment. Please refer to the discussion of Mood Disorder Due to a General Medical Condition on pages 25–26 of the User's Guide and Substance-Induced Mood Disorder on pages 26–27 of the User's Guide for a detailed discussion of how to evaluate these criteria.

Ratings for Psychotic Disorder NOS (item C39)

This is the place to diagnose any Psychotic Disorder that does not meet the criteria for the specific Psychotic Disorders described earlier. There are several examples given, but the most frequent reason for using this category in the SCID-CV is that you know the patient has had psychotic symptoms, but you do not have enough information to make a more specific diagnosis. This category also applies to the brief psychotic experiences that can occur in some patients with Borderline Personality Disorder when they are subjected to extreme stress.

9.6 Module D. Mood Disorders

Whereas Module A was for rating *Mood Episodes*, this module is for recording *Mood Disorder* diagnoses (other than Dysthymic Disorder, Mood Disorder Due to a General Medical Condition, and Substance-Induced Mood Disorder). These are Bipolar I Disorder, Bipolar II Disorder, Other Bipolar Disorder (which includes Cyclothymic Disorder and Bipolar Disorder NOS), Major Depressive Disorder, and Depressive Disorder NOS. As in Module C, the task in this module is to evaluate whether the specific criteria for Mood Disorders are met based on information gathered in Modules A, B, and C. Going through this module is akin to following the DSM-IV decision tree for Mood Disorders (pages 696–697 in DSM-IV).

Ratings for Bipolar I and Bipolar II Disorder (items D1–D9)

The minimum requirement for a diagnosis of Bipolar I Disorder is a Manic or Mixed Episode that is not due to a substance or general medical condition, is not already part of a diagnosis of Schizoaffective Disorder, and is not superimposed on a chronic Psychotic Disorder (which would have been diagnosed in Module C). The minimum requirement for a diagnosis of Bipolar II Disorder is one Hypomanic AND one Major Depressive Episode, neither due to a substance or general medical condition. Bipolar II cannot be diagnosed if there has ever been a Manic or Mixed Episode. The question may arise as to how the clinician is to know whether there have been any Mixed Episodes, since Module A does not include ratings for a Mixed Episode—only for Major Depressive, Manic, or Hypomanic Episodes. This issue is actually diagnostically relevant only for determining the type of the current episode—past Mixed Episodes are not distinguished in the SCID-CV from past Manic Episodes because the presence of either type warrants a lifetime diagnosis of Bipolar I Disorder. The current episode is considered to be Mixed if BOTH a current Major Depressive and current Manic Episode are coded "+" in Module A and it is determined that the criteria have been met for both *nearly every day* for at least a 1-week period. If a current Manic Episode is present but the criteria have not been met for a current Major Depressive Episode, the clinician should go back and consider whether the criteria for a Major Depressive Episode have been met for at least 1 week, in which case the current episode type for the Bipolar I Disorder would be Mixed.

Ratings for Other Bipolar Disorders (items D10–D12)

If criteria are not met for either Bipolar I or Bipolar II Disorder AND there are clinically significant manic or hypomanic symptoms that are not better accounted for by a Psychotic Disorder, then a diagnosis of Cyclothymic Disorder or another "bipolar spectrum disorder" may be warranted. Note that before one of these disorders can be considered, the clinician must first rule out a general medical condition or a substance as the cause of the manic symptoms (see pages 10–12 and 24–27 in the User's Guide for a discussion of this process).

Ratings for Major Depressive Disorder (items D13–D16)

The diagnosis of Major Depressive Disorder requires a minimum of one Major Depressive Episode that is not due to a general medical condition or substance, is not already included in

a diagnosis of Schizoaffective Disorder, and is not superimposed on a chronic Psychotic Disorder (which would have already been diagnosed in Module C). Note that for Major Depressive Disorder to be considered recurrent, one needs only to determine that there was a period lasting at least 2 months in which the depressive symptomatology consistently fell below the five-symptom threshold for a Major Depressive Episode—*not* a 2-month period of full remission.

Ratings for Depressive Disorder NOS (items D17–D19)

If criteria are not met for Major Depressive Disorder, Dysthymic Disorder, or Adjustment Disorder *and* there are clinically significant depressive symptoms that are not due to the direct physiological effects of a general medical condition or substance use, then a diagnosis of Depressive Disorder Not Otherwise Specified may be warranted.

9.7 Module E. Substance Use Disorders

Module E contains ratings for the Substance Use Disorders (Dependence and Abuse), which cover problems caused by the patient's pattern of substance use. Psychiatric symptoms (e.g., psychosis, depression, anxiety) related to the direct effects of the substance on the central nervous system are diagnosed as Substance-Induced Disorders and are located throughout the SCID-CV according to the type of symptom presentation (i.e., Substance-Induced Mood Disorder in Module A, Substance-Induced Psychotic Disorder in Module C, and Substance-Induced Anxiety Disorder in Module F). The SCID-CV separates the evaluation of Alcohol from other substances because it is legal, more widely used than other substances, and most users do not have problems with it.

Procedure for Rating Alcohol Use Disorders

The Alcohol section begins with a series of screening questions to determine whether the patient's pattern of alcohol use is substantial enough to warrant a detailed evaluation of Alcohol Dependence and Abuse or if the patient's use of alcohol is insignificant and does not require further assessment. Because patients often minimize (or underestimate) their drinking habits, the clinician should skip the Alcohol section *only* if there is absolutely no question that there have never been any incidents of excessive drinking or alcohol-related problems. Because the definition of Alcohol Abuse requires *recurrent* problems associated with alcohol, infrequent but nonetheless heavy drinking may still warrant a diagnosis of Alcohol Abuse. As a rule of thumb, if the patient reports ever having had five or more drinks at any one time, acknowledges ever having a problem related to drinking, or admits that others have objected to his or her drinking, then the Alcohol Use Disorders section of the SCID-CV should be explored.

Because a diagnosis of Alcohol Abuse is relevant only for those individuals whose pattern of use does *not* meet the criteria for Alcohol Dependence, it might seem to make sense to ask the questions for Dependence first. However, because it is expected that the majority of individuals who screen positive with these low threshold screening questions will not have Alcohol Dependence, the SCID-CV first checks the four criteria for Alcohol Abuse. If the criteria are met for Abuse, then and only then is the assessment of the seven criteria for Dependence required. However, if information from the Overview and alcohol screening questions suggests that a diagnosis of Alcohol Dependence is likely, the clinician should start with the questions for Alcohol Dependence (item E7) because, if the criteria are met for Dependence, Alcohol Abuse need not be assessed. This design minimizes the total number of substance-related questions that have to be asked— four questions for the majority who have had as many as five drinks on one occasion but have never had an Alcohol Use Disorder, seven questions for those most likely to have Dependence, and eleven questions for those few in the middle (i.e., for those patients who admit to having some problems with alcohol but not enough to suspect Dependence, the clinician starts with the four Abuse questions; if the criteria are met for Abuse, the clinician must then follow up with the seven questions for Dependence).

Procedure for Rating Nonalcohol Substance Use Disorders

The initial task is to identify the one drug class (if any) most likely to have been associated with a Nonalcohol Substance Use Disorder. This section therefore begins with an inquiry about the level of drug use for each drug class. The procedure for using this section is as follows. Give the patient the drug list (the last page of the SCID-CV Scoresheet) and ask which drugs he or she has ever tried. Note that the list of drugs given to the patient matches the list of drugs on page 43 of the Scoresheet. For each of those acknowledged, the clinician should identify the period of heaviest use and the pattern of use during that time and record this information on page 43 of the Scoresheet. After selecting the drug class that was used the most or caused the most problems, the clinician must choose one of the following three options: 1) to proceed directly to the evaluation of Substance Dependence if the level of drug use or the presence of substance-related problems indicates that Dependence is likely; 2) to proceed with the evaluation of Substance Abuse if the level of drug use is such that Dependence is unlikely (a guideline suggested in the Research Version of the SCID is that Dependence is unlikely if the patient has never used the drug more than 10 times in any 1-month period); or 3) to skip the evaluation of a nonalcohol substance use disorder if there is no possibility of a substance problem (e.g., if the patient has never used any drug or tried a drug only one time). Note that if option 2 is chosen and the criteria are met for Abuse, the clinician must then check to see if the criteria have also been met for Dependence for that drug (in which case only the diagnosis of Substance Dependence is given). Note also that a diagnosis of Substance Abuse or Substance Dependence may also apply to prescribed medication if the patient has had a history of taking more than was prescribed.

Ratings for Alcohol/Other Substance Abuse (items E2–E6 and E18–E22)

Although rated separately in the SCID-CV, the Abuse items are identical for Alcohol and other drugs. A rating of "+" on any of the Abuse items generally depends on the patient's recognizing the problem and telling you about it. A patient who regularly has a few beers, a few martinis, or even a few puffs of marijuana with lunch, but denies that it has ever caused problems, cannot be diagnosed with Substance Abuse. If you suspect that the patient is minimizing the consequences of drinking or using drugs you may need to gently confront his or her denial (e.g., "It's hard for me to imagine that being stoned while working on a roof wasn't dangerous. Are you sure you were functioning as well as you do when you're not stoned?"). Interviewing informants is often crucial to the accurate assessment of Substance Abuse and Dependence.

Note that the problems listed in the criteria must occur repeatedly to be coded "+"—at least twice in a 12-month period. One arrest for driving while intoxicated does not count (although it is likely anyone who gets stopped for drunk driving has had other times when he or she drove while intoxicated and was not caught, in which case criterion A(2) would be coded "+").

Criterion A(1) (items E2 and E18). A rating of "+" for this item requires specific evidence that it was the effects of the substance use that resulted in the patient's failure to fulfill a major role obligation on at least two occasions.

Criterion A(2) (items E3 and E19). A common error in rating this item is to be overinclusive and assume that any level of substance use in a situation that requires alertness would qualify. The item should be rated "+" only when the substance use causes sufficient impairment to create a physically hazardous condition (e.g., driving or hunting while intoxicated). Note that the question in parentheses asks the patient to judge how impaired he or she was when driving (or doing any other potentially dangerous activity). You may give the benefit of the doubt to someone who says, for example, that he can drive perfectly well after having two beers.

Although getting drunk or stoned and walking home through a dangerous neighborhood or having unprotected sex with someone the patient does not know well while intoxicated is certainly risky, neither would warrant a rating of "+"—the intent of this item is to rate behavior that puts the patient in immediate danger because his or her coordination or cognition is impaired by the substance.

Criterion A(3) (items E4 and E20). This item should be rated "+" only if the legal problems are a direct consequence of the effects of the substance (e.g., arrest for violent behavior resulting from intoxication). Legal problems resulting from procurement or possession of illicit substances do not count because these are so much a function of local laws, attitudes, and enforcement policies.

Criterion A(4) (items E5 and E21). This item is difficult to evaluate when the interpersonal conflict is possibly attributable to a relational problem rather than to a problem with the patient's substance use. For example, arguments about occasional nonproblematic substance use that are initiated by a spouse who believes any drinking is wrong would not warrant a rating of "+."

Ratings for Alcohol/Other Substance Dependence (items E7–E14, and E23–E30)

The criteria have been reordered from DSM-IV to make them more user-friendly.

Criterion A(3) (items E7 and E23). The intent of this item is to capture the patient's failed attempts to put some limits on his or her drinking (e.g., "I'll just have a few beers and then go home" or "I'll stop at the bar for only half an hour"). Note that the breaking of these self-imposed limits (e.g., the patient ends up drinking a couple of six-packs or staying in the bar for hours) must occur *often* to be coded "+." There is something of a paradox inherent in the evaluation of this item (and criterion A(4) as well). To qualify for these items, the patient must have developed enough insight about having a substance problem to want to control its use. These items are, therefore, impossible to evaluate in someone who has a very heavy pattern of use but denies any need to control or cut down use. For example, heavy users of cannabis may be unlikely to attempt to cut down or control their use of the substance because of their perception that cannabis is harmless.

Criterion A(4) (items E8 and E24). This item describes unsuccessful attempts to cut down or control drinking or drug use over a longer period of time—weeks, months, or years—as opposed to planning for an evening's drinking or drug use.

Criterion A(5) (items E9 and E25). This three-part item covers the various ways in which drinking or drug use may become a central focus of the patient's life. It is especially variable across the classes of drugs because of differences in cost, availability, legality, and typical pattern of use of the particular substance. For example, the high cost, daily need, and relative unavailability of opioids is much more likely to result in a patient becoming totally preoccupied with the daily task of procuring them. In contrast, this item is less likely to apply to inhalants because of the low cost, wide availability in stores, and typical pattern of intermittent use.

Criterion A(6) (items E10 and E26). The prototype for this item is a street-corner alcoholic who has essentially given up all activities except those associated with drinking. It may also be applied, for example, to an amateur athlete who has stopped doing sports because of substance use, or a person who has stopped seeing all his good friends and now hangs out with a group of heavy drug users.

Criterion A(7) (items E11 and E27). This item is meant to tap a pattern of compulsive use of the substance and does not refer merely to the adverse physical or psychological consequences of using the substance. To qualify for a rating of "+" on this item, the patient must understand that the physical or psychological problems are a result of the substance and still be unable to stop using or cut down significantly. Examples of physical problems include cirrhosis caused by alcohol, damage to nasal mucosa from sniffing cocaine, and so on. Examples of psychological problems are alcohol-induced pugnacity that leads to frequent fights, cocaine-induced paranoia, or panic attacks precipitated by marijuana.

The most frequent noxious physical effect of alcohol is a hangover. When hangovers are severe and frequent, and the patient still continues to drink, a coding of "+" is justified on this item.

Criterion A(1) (items E12 and E28). Anyone who drinks develops some tolerance from the time they were an adolescent experimenting with alcohol. This item is meant to capture those whose tolerance increased markedly from the time they began drinking fairly regularly to some later time (e.g., "I used to get drunk on three beers. Now I can drink two six-packs and not be drunk."). The development of tolerance occurs most frequently with alcohol, amphetamine, cocaine, nicotine, opioids, and sedatives (especially barbiturates). Tolerance for many drugs (e.g., cocaine, barbiturates, heroin) is usually apparent to the patient. For drugs such as marijuana, where the quality of the drug varies markedly, it may not be possible to establish tolerance.

Criterion A(2) (items E13 and E29). Withdrawal is indicated by the development of the charac-

teristic substance-specific withdrawal syndrome shortly after stopping or decreasing the amount of the substance. In some cases, the patient never allows the withdrawal syndrome to develop because he or she starts taking more of the substance in anticipation of the onset of withdrawal symptoms. The severity and clinical significance of the withdrawal syndrome vary by class of substance. Characteristic withdrawal syndromes are most apparent with alcohol, sedatives, and opioids. Criteria sets are also provided for withdrawal from amphetamine and cocaine. Although withdrawal symptoms sometimes occur, no specific criteria sets are provided for withdrawal from cannabis, hallucinogens, inhalants, or PCP.

9.8 Module F. Anxiety and Other Disorders

Ratings for Panic Disorder (items F1–F24)

Criterion A(1) (item F1). The term "panic attack" is often incorrectly used by patients to describe any escalating anxiety, but the hallmark of a true panic attack is the sudden and intense onset of symptoms. The physical symptoms and terror are often overwhelming, and initial panic attacks may lead a patient to seek emergency care because of concerns that he or she may be having a heart attack.

The presence of a panic attack is not necessarily indicative of Panic Disorder because panic attacks can occur in the context of a number of Anxiety Disorders. For example, if a person with a snake phobia goes on a hike and has a panic attack after accidentally stepping on a snake, this would not warrant an additional diagnosis of Panic Disorder. By definition, *at least two* of the panic attacks in Panic Disorder must have been "unexpected." Assessing whether a panic attack was "unexpected" may be difficult because patients with Panic Disorder commonly (and mistakenly) believe that there is a cause-and-effect relationship between the situations in which the attacks have developed and the attacks themselves. For example, a patient who experienced several unexpected attacks while shopping may assume that it was the experience of being in a crowded store that led to the attacks and therefore not consider the attack to be "unexpected." In such a situation, the clinician should use the follow-up question, "Have you *ever* had a panic attack when you didn't expect to?" or "When you were in the store, right before you had your first attack, were you already feeling anxious or were you feeling OK?"

For some patients, attacks occur following a frightening thought, such as worrying that something terrible will happen to them or to a loved one. Such attacks should still be regarded as "unexpected" because the concept of "unexpected" refers to the absence of a clear association between an *environmental* stimulus and the occurrence of the panic attack. Common sense (we hope) will lead the clinician not to include as "unexpected" panic attacks that occur in response to unexpected but realistic dangers, such as being mugged. Similarly, panic attacks that occur in response to delusions about being harmed should not be regarded as "unexpected."

Criterion A(2) (item F2).   The diagnosis of Panic Disorder requires that at least one of the panic attacks be clinically significant. The three subparts of this criterion present three different ways in which clinical significance may be manifested: 1) persistent worry about the implications of the attack (e.g., that the attack means the patient is going crazy or suffering from a medical illness); 2) worry about having additional attacks; or 3) a change in lifestyle (most commonly, avoidance of situations or activities or modifications to accommodate the attack, such as always being near an exit, sitting on the aisle of a theater, etc.). Patients who have had panic attacks but are not particularly bothered by them would warrant a rating of "–" for this item.

Criteria for Panic Attack (items F3–F17).   In DSM-IV, panic attack is defined using a freestanding criteria set that is not part of the criteria set for Panic Disorder per se. The SCID-CV embeds the evaluation of whether the discrete episode of symptoms constitutes a true panic attack or just a limited symptom attack (i.e., less than four symptoms) in the evaluation of Panic Disorder.

Before presenting the 13 symptoms of a panic attack to the patient, the clinician is instructed to first inquire about the most recent panic attack in an open-ended way (i.e., "When was the last bad one? What was the first thing you noticed?" etc.). This allows the patient an opportunity to describe the attack in his or her own words, which is helpful in determining whether the experience has the qualities of a true panic attack. This method is also helpful in encouraging

the patient to focus on a single specific attack when endorsing the characteristic symptoms. Note that if fewer than four symptoms are endorsed, the clinician should ask the patient whether he or she has had attacks during which there were more symptoms. If so, the clinician should go back and reapply the list of 13 symptoms to this more severe attack and then confirm that such attacks have occurred repeatedly.

The requirement that the symptoms reach a peak within 10 minutes is to differentiate a panic attack from slowly escalating anxiety. In fact, panic attacks often peak within seconds and almost always within a few minutes. Although most panic attacks subside within an hour, some patients may continue to have symptoms and a high level of anxiety for hours after the peak.

Criterion C (item F18).   This criterion instructs the clinician to consider and rule out a general medical condition or a substance as an etiological factor for the panic attacks. Remember to carefully assess caffeine intake, and remember that caffeine is present in a variety of foods and over-the-counter medications like Anacin. Although substance use may be associated with the *initial onset* of panic attacks, a substance use etiology should be considered when subsequent panic attacks occur *only* in the context of substance use. See pages 10–12 (in the User's Guide) for a general discussion of how to apply this criterion and pages 24–27 (in the User's Guide) for a discussion of the criteria for a Mood Disorder Due to a General Medical Condition and a Substance-Induced Mood Disorder, which also apply to Anxiety Disorder Due to a General Medical Condition and Substance-Induced Anxiety Disorder.

Criterion D (item F19).   This criterion asks the clinician to consider whether the panic attacks are better accounted for by another mental disorder. The judgment depends on determining whether the panic attacks are cued by an anxiety-provoking stimulus arising in the context of another disorder. For example, consider a patient with long-standing Social Phobia who has a panic attack while speaking in front of a large group of people. Since the panic attack was triggered by exposure to an anxiety-provoking situation (e.g., speaking in public) it is considered to be better accounted for by Social Phobia. Similarly, if someone with Posttraumatic Stress Disorder develops a panic attack when exposed to a stimulus that reminds the person of the traumatic event, then the attack would not be considered a symptom of Panic Disorder. Note that this criterion does NOT set up a strict hierarchy between Panic Disorder and other mental disorders (i.e., DSM-IV does not instruct you NOT to diagnose Panic Disorder if the attacks occur during another disorder). Instead, clinical judgment is required to determine whether the other disorder "better accounts for" the panic attacks. The clinician may need to set aside the evaluation of this criterion pending completion of the remainder of the SCID-CV if it seems likely that another disorder that accounts for the panic attacks may be present.

Criterion B: Agoraphobia. Some patients with Panic Disorder manage to grit their teeth and suffer panic attacks without developing any avoidance behavior, but most begin to associate certain situations with their panic attacks and consequently avoid those situations (or else endure them only with great anxiety). This avoidance may range from simply not driving a car because the patient is afraid of having an attack while driving to never leaving home because of fears of having an attack in a place that is not "safe."

Criterion B(1) (item F20). To rate this item "+," the patient should report that a situation is avoided because of fears that a panic attack is more likely to develop in that situation or that escape from the situation may be difficult or embarrassing in case of having a panic attack. In some cases, the patient may not be aware of the reason certain situations are avoided. If the avoidance develops soon after the onset of panic attacks, the clinician may infer that the avoidance is related to the panic attacks.

Criterion B(2) (item F21). Note that a rating of "+" may still be appropriate for a patient who is able to force himself or herself to go into the agoraphobic situations as long as there is either marked distress or the need for a companion to accompany the patient.

Criterion B(3) (item F22). This criterion is similar to criterion D in Panic Disorder in that it reminds the clinician to consider whether the fear and avoidance may be better characterized as part of another mental disorder. Two of the most difficult boundaries are with Specific Phobia and Social Phobia. Typically, Agoraphobia involves avoidance of a cluster of situations, reflecting the general unpredictability of panic attacks. In contrast, a Specific Phobia tends to be limited to one consistently feared situation. Furthermore, the onset of Agoraphobia is related to the onset of panic attacks, whereas Specific Phobias tend to be either lifelong or related to a traumatic experience. Determining whether avoidance of social situations is related to Social Phobia or to fear of developing a panic attack in a social situation (which would warrant a diagnosis of Agoraphobia) generally depends on determining the temporal relationship between the onset of panic attacks and the social avoidance. If a patient develops social avoidance only *after* the onset of panic attacks, then Agoraphobia is the most appropriate diagnosis. A patient with long-standing social avoidance who develops panic attacks only when in social situations would be considered to have Social Phobia. Note that this criterion does *not* preclude making a diagnosis of *both* Panic Disorder With Agoraphobia and another disorder characterized by avoidance in the same patient (e.g., a patient with a long-standing dog phobia since childhood who develops unexpected panic attacks in situations without the presence of dogs).

Ratings for Obsessive-Compulsive Disorder (items F25–F38)

Criterion A: Obsessions (items F25–F29). The most common diagnostic problem is distinguishing true obsessions from other repetitive distressing thoughts, such as excessive worries about realistic concerns, depressive ruminations, and delusions. Obsessions have an intrusive, inappropriate, and "ego-alien" quality and are experienced by the patient as something different and stranger than the worries or preoccupations that characterize Generalized Anxiety Disorder or a normal reaction to life's unpredictability. The recurrent, intrusive, and anxiety-provoking thought, while driving, that one ran over a small child without realizing it, is an obsession. Spending an equal amount of time worrying about one's retirement is more likely to be an aspect of Generalized Anxiety Disorder. Unlike obsessions, depressive ruminations and delusions are generally not perceived as intrusive or inappropriate but are understood by the patient as a valid focus of concern, even if he or she realizes that the concern is excessive and tries to stop thinking about it.

In those situations when the differential diagnosis is particularly challenging, it may be useful to remember the fact that obsessions and compulsions usually go together (in fact, 90% of the time, according to the DSM-IV Obsessive-Compulsive Disorder field trial). Therefore, in trying to distinguish between an Obsessive-Compulsive Disorder obsession and other repetitive thoughts, the clinching point may be whether compulsions are also present.

Criterion A: Compulsions (items F30–F33). Compulsions are distinguished from other forms of repetitive behavior by the underlying motivation for the behavior—to reduce or prevent the anxiety associated with an obsession. For example, hand washing alleviates the anxiety triggered by the obsession that one is contaminated; repeating a prayer exactly 36 times is meant to counteract the distress caused by having an obsessive obscene thought. Determining that the behavior is intended to reduce the anxiety accompanying an obsession is helpful in differentiating a compulsion from other repetitive behaviors such as tics and stereotypies. The most common compulsions are behaviors such as hand washing, repetitive touching, or picking up and replacing an object repetitively, or mental acts such as counting or repeating a word or phrase.

Criterion B (item F34). The prototypical patient with Obsessive-Compulsive Disorder is aware that his or her obsessions and compulsions are unreasonable (e.g., that it is ridiculous to be concerned about contamination from germs that might arise from touching newspapers). Over time, some patients with Obsessive-Compulsive Disorder lose insight as to the excessive nature of their obsessive concerns or compulsive behaviors and may, in a later stage of the illness, describe the obsessions or compulsions as being reasonable. For such patients, it is essential to establish whether *at some time in the past* (usually early in the course of the illness) the obsessions and compulsions were regarded as unreasonable (e.g., "when the hand washing first started, did you feel that you were washing your hands much more than you should or than really made sense?").

Criterion C (item F35). This criterion requires that the obsessions or compulsions be clinically significant. Note that the standard DSM-IV clinical significance criterion is augmented by a phrase indicating that the obsessions or compulsions may be "time consuming (take more than an hour a day)." This clause allows the clinician to

conclude that impairment is present even in the face of the patient's apparent lack of concern about the behavior or the rationalization that it is useful.

Criterion D (item F36). An additional diagnosis of Obsessive-Compulsive Disorder should not be given with another mental disorder if the repetitive thoughts or behaviors can be considered to be features of the other mental disorder. Most of the examples of symptoms of other disorders that are given in the SCID-CV do not really meet the test of "intrusive and inappropriate." For example, when a patient with Anorexia Nervosa is preoccupied with measuring the exact number of calories in the food she eats, she may agree only that it is excessive, not foolish. However, if the obsessions or compulsions are clearly symptoms of another disorder, the clinician may skip out of the diagnosis of Obsessive-Compulsive Disorder without spending a lot of time deciding whether the symptoms are intrusive and inappropriate or just excessive. (Of course, Anorexia Nervosa does not protect someone against Obsessive-Compulsive Disorder; the patient with Anorexia Nervosa may also have hand-washing rituals that are unrelated to the eating disorder and therefore be given both diagnoses.)

Criterion E (item F37). Obsessive-Compulsive Disorder is rarely a result of a general medical condition or substance use.

Common Pitfall. Neophyte SCIDers may become obsessively concerned with the precise meaning of each word in the definitions and assign a diagnosis to a patient who does not warrant it. Many people have some obsessive thoughts or compulsive behavior, but Obsessive-Compulsive Disorder is a severe and relatively infrequent condition.

Ratings for Posttraumatic Stress Disorder (items F39–F64)

Record of Traumatic Events (item F39). The evaluation of Posttraumatic Stress Disorder begins with a screen that first reviews the individual's lifetime history of exposure to severely traumatic experiences and then determines whether any of these traumatic experiences have been reexperienced in the form of dreams, flashbacks, intrusive thoughts, or strong reactions when in situations that are reminiscent of the trauma. If so, the clinician should proceed with the evaluation of Posttraumatic Stress Disorder, focusing on the event identified in the screen. If more than one traumatic experience is reported, the clinician should ask the patient to choose the one that seems to have affected him or her the most. If, during the evaluation of Posttraumatic Stress Disorder for this particular stressor, it becomes clear that the criteria for Posttraumatic Stress Disorder are not being met, the clinician should determine whether one of the other stressors may have had a greater impact on the patient and then reevaluate the criteria in relation to this different stressor.

Criterion A(1) (item F40). In evaluating whether a stressor qualifies as a potential source of Posttraumatic Stress Disorder, both the type of stressor ("actual or threatened death or serious injury or threat to the physical integrity of self or others") and the context of exposure ("experienced, witnessed, or confronted with") should be considered. In DSM-IV, stressors are limited to events that pose a threat to life, limb, or physical integrity. Stressors that, while distressing, are not life threatening (e.g., being humiliated by a boss at the office) do not warrant a rating of "+" for this item. Although the prototypical stressor for Posttraumatic Stress Disorder is a wartime combat experience, the concept also includes other life-threatening experiences such as being a victim of a serious crime, accident, or disaster. The phrase "threat to physical integrity" includes all experiences of sexual assault or sexual molestation, not just those in which the victim perceives a threat of violence. The context of the exposure includes having one's life threatened; having the direct personal experience of seeing someone else being threatened, injured, or killed; or hearing the news of a loved one being hurt or killed. It is not meant to include more indirect and impersonal experiences such as hearing a news report of a catastrophe occurring to strangers. Similarly, the expected death of a loved one of natural causes at an advanced age does not qualify as a Posttraumatic Stress Disorder stressor.

Criterion A(2) (item F41). This criterion requires that the patient be profoundly affected by the stressor and react to it with extreme feelings of "fear, helplessness, or horror." Children are less likely to articulate their feelings, and this item may be inferred by a change in their behavior.

Criterion B (items F42–F47). The reexperiencing of the traumatic event can occur spontaneously (intrusive memories, flashbacks, or dreams) or can be triggered by a wide variety of stimuli that remind the patient of the traumatic event. For example, smoke from a campfire may produce profound terror in someone who has been trapped in a house fire. Flashbacks to wartime may be triggered by loud noises, seeing war movies, or tropical rainstorms. In some cases, the trigger may be a symbolic representation of the actual stimulus (e.g., a policeman for a concentration camp survivor). Occasionally, it may be difficult to differentiate a flashback from a psychotic experience. In contrast with psychotic symptoms, the sense that one is reliving the traumatic experience in Posttraumatic Stress Disorder is transient, self-limited, and understandable in the context of the exposure to the prior stressor. Note that the reexperiencing must be persistent—a few nightmares or intrusive memories do not satisfy this criterion.

Criteria C and D (items F48–F61). These criteria include symptoms that are much less specific than those in A and B, and are seen in many other disorders. Many people, for instance, try to avoid talking or thinking about bad things that have happened to them, whether or not the bad things were traumatic. Diminished interest, detachment, a restricted range of affect, insomnia, difficulty concentrating, and so on may be symptoms of a Depressive Disorder or of a Personality Disorder. It is important that the clinician clarify that the symptoms in C and D developed after the trauma. (In the case of a childhood trauma, it is impossible to know what the person would be like had he or she not had the experience. Following the SCID principle that one does not make a diagnosis without the evidence, we would be hesitant to diagnose Posttraumatic Stress Disorder in an adult who has had the symptoms as long as he or she can remember.)

Criterion E (item F62). The minimum duration requirement for a diagnosis of Posttraumatic Stress Disorder is 1 month. For extreme reactions to extreme stressors lasting for less than 1 month, consider a diagnosis of Acute Stress Disorder (a new disorder added to DSM-IV, pages 429–432).

Criterion F (item F63). If, at this point in the interview, you have any doubt about whether the syndrome causes significant distress or impairment, it probably does not.

Ratings for Other Anxiety, Somatoform, and Eating Disorders (F65–F76)

The remaining disorders in this section (except Adjustment Disorder) are presented in a summarized format. To the left of each description is a screening question (taken from the Research Version of the SCID) that serves to help the clinician determine if there is any evidence suggesting that the disorder might be present. If the patient answers "yes" to the screening question, the clinician should refer to the diagnostic criteria in DSM-IV to determine whether the diagnosis should be made. Note that these disorders are evaluated in their entirety in the Research Version of the SCID. Interested clinicians should contact Biometrics Research (212) 960-5524 for further information.

Agoraphobia Without History of Panic Disorder (AWOPD) (item F65). This disorder is similar to Panic Disorder With Agoraphobia, but the concern is about panic-like symptoms as opposed to full-blown panic attacks. In Panic Disorder *With* Agoraphobia, there is anxiety about being in places or situations from which escape may be difficult or embarrassing if a panic attack occurs. In this condition (AWOPD), the anxiety is focused on being in places or situations from which escape may be difficult or embarrassing in the event of having panic-like symptoms (either a specific uncontrollable symptom such as loss of bowel control or else subthreshold versions of panic attacks known as "limited symptom attacks").

Social Phobia (item F66) and Specific Phobia (item F67). There is a wide range of social triggers that may be associated with a diagnosis of Social Phobia—what they all have in common is that the patient fears acting in a way that will be humiliating or embarrassing. Some people are afraid of any kind of scrutiny—they choose to work by themselves, will not go to parties, or will not go out on dates because they are extremely self-conscious and believe that others will judge them to be foolish, stupid, or inept. Other socially phobic patients are comfortable in interpersonal situations but uncomfortable about various situations in which they are required to "perform." This more circumscribed form of Social Phobia includes traditional performance situations such as public speaking or playing a musical instrument in public, as well as other behaviors that are only a performance in the person's mind: fears about

urinating in a public bathroom, writing in front of others, or eating in front of others. A diagnosis of Specific Phobia applies to circumscribed objects or situations (other than social) that are avoided or else endured with excessive anxiety. The hallmark characteristic of a phobia is that the fear is way out of proportion to the degree of realistic danger posed by the object or situation.

A diagnosis of Social or Specific Phobia is not made unless the avoidance, anticipatory anxiety, or distress is clinically significant (i.e., interferes with functioning, social activities, or relationships, or if there is marked distress *about* having the phobia). Thus, for example, a public speaking phobia in a plumber who is almost never called on to address groups of people is unlikely to meet the criterion, as is a snake phobia in someone who rarely leaves New York City. Some individuals who seriously constrict their lives to avoid social (or other phobic) situations may report a lack of distress because their phobias are never activated. A diagnosis of Social or Specific Phobia may still be justified if the clinician judges that the phobia has a significant negative impact on the patient's functioning.

Generalized Anxiety Disorder (item F68). This disorder describes the person who may be known by acquaintances as a "worry wart." The anxiety or worry is not focused on one or two issues but is panoramic. For example, a patient with Generalized Anxiety Disorder might worry about the safety of her children, the possibility of being late for appointments, not having enough time to finish a project, what to wear to a party, whether her job is in jeopardy, whether there are jellyfish in the water, and so on. She worries much of the time, and everyone she knows thinks it is excessive.

Anxiety Disorder Not Otherwise Specified (items F69–F71). This residual diagnosis applies to presentations characterized by anxiety that do not meet the criteria for a specific Anxiety or Mood Disorder or an Adjustment Disorder and that are not caused by the direct physiological effects of a general medical condition or substance.

Somatization Disorder/Undifferentiated Somatoform Disorder (item F72). These diagnoses are for presentations characterized by the presence of one or more "somatoform" symptoms (i.e., physical symptoms that suggest a physical illness but are not fully explained by a general medical condition, by the direct effects of a substance, or as a culturally sanctioned behavior or experience). Somatization Disorder and Undifferentiated Somatoform Disorder differ based on the number of required somatoform symptoms. Somatization Disorder requires a pattern of somatoform symptoms consisting of at least *one* pseudoneurological symptom, pain symptoms in at least *four* different anatomical sites, *two* gastrointestinal symptoms, and *one* sexual symptom. Undifferentiated Somatoform Disorder is for presentation of one (or more) somatoform symptoms that last at least 6 months.

Hypochondriasis (item F73). The essential feature of Hypochondriasis is preoccupation with the fear of having, or the belief that one has, a serious disease. This is in contrast with the other Somatoform Disorders in which the patient's primary focus is on the physical symptom itself. As with the other Somatoform Disorders, it is important to make sure that the patient has had an *appropriate* medical evaluation before assuming that the preoccupation is unwarranted.

Body Dysmorphic Disorder (item F74). The evaluation of Body Dysmorphic Disorder is generally more straightforward than the evaluation of the other Somatoform Disorders because the pathological nature of the patient's concern about appearance does not usually require a medical evaluation. However, in some cases the boundary between this disorder and "normal" concerns or dissatisfactions about appearance can be difficult to discern. The diagnosis should be reserved for those who become preoccupied by their supposed deformity or are tormented by it.

Anorexia Nervosa (item F75). Although abnormally low weight is necessary for a diagnosis of Anorexia Nervosa, it is not sufficient. There must be evidence that the person is underweight because of a "refusal" to maintain a normal body weight.

Bulimia Nervosa (item F76). A diagnosis of Bulimia Nervosa requires both regular binge eating and the use of inappropriate mechanisms to counteract the weight-gaining effects of the binges. Binge eating occurs during a discrete period of time, involves consuming a huge number of calories, and is characterized by the sense of having lost control. The most common of these compensatory behaviors is some form of purging (self-induced vomiting or laxative abuse). Less common compensatory behaviors include fasting, excessive exercise, and manipulation of insulin dose by patients with diabetes.

Ratings for Adjustment Disorder (items F77–F82)

In most cases, this section is skipped during the administration of the SCID-CV because another more specific diagnosis has been made. The clinician needs to consider this disorder only if there is a current problem described in the Overview, but no other Axis I disorder has been identified by the SCID-CV to account for it. The border between Adjustment Disorder and ordinary problems of life may be clarified by the notion that Adjustment Disorder implies that the severity of the disturbance is sufficient to justify clinical attention or treatment.

10. Training

Ideally, training should involve the following sequence:

1. Study the Basic Features, Conventions and Usage, and DOs and DON'Ts sections in this manual, with the SCID-CV alongside.

2. Carefully read through every word of the SCID-CV, making sure that you understand all of the instructions, the questions, and the diagnostic criteria. As you are reading through each module, refer to the corresponding User's Guide section of Special Instructions for Individual Modules. Review the Diagnostic Features and Differential Diagnosis sections of DSM-IV text for those disorders included in the SCID-CV.

3. Practice reading the SCID-CV questions aloud so that eventually it sounds as if SCID-CV is your mother tongue.

4. Try out the SCID-CV with a colleague (or significant other) who can assume the role of a patient.

5. Watch the SCID-101 videotape training program. Videotapes are available from Biometrics Research (212) 960-5524.

6. Role-play the cases (see Appendix) with a colleague. These have been designed to take you

through the SCID-CV modules, not necessarily to demonstrate your dramatic talent.

7. Try out the SCID-CV on actual patients with other clinicians who are learning how to use the SCID-CV, by observing the interview and making independent ratings. This should be followed by a discussion of the interviewing technique and sources of disagreement in the ratings.

8. Finally, we list the four most common errors of new SCIDers to emphasize the areas to which you should pay special attention:
   a) The description of behavior or symptoms is insufficient to rate the criterion "+" or "−."
   b) The clinician mistakenly circles a "−" for an exclusion criterion, resulting in a trip to the wrong section of the SCID-CV.
   c) The clinician fails to follow the skip-out instructions and therefore ends up in the wrong section of the SCID-CV.
   d) The overview is too skimpy or too unfocused (and therefore LONG) to enable the clinician to make diagnostic hypotheses with any confidence.

9. The best way to become comfortable and efficient with the SCID-CV is to PRACTICE, PRACTICE, PRACTICE! This reduces the administration time, improves clinical skills, and enhances the reliability and validity of the measure.

11. Reliability and Validity

Traditionally, assessment instruments are presented with data supporting their "reliability" and "validity." Reliability for diagnostic assessment instruments is generally evaluated by comparing the agreement among independent evaluations by two or more interviewers across a group of subjects. The results are usually reported with a statistic, kappa, that takes into account agreement caused by chance (Spitzer et al. 1967). Because the SCID-CV is a not a fully structured interview and requires the clinical judgment of the interviewer, the reliability of the SCID-CV is a function of the particular circumstances in which it is being used.

Using an earlier version of the Axis I SCID, data were collected on 506 pairs of interviews at six sites in a test-retest reliability study (Williams et al. 1992). A very stringent test of the SCID was conducted in which the subjects were selected randomly and the interviewers had no access to charts or treatment staff. The kappas for the Axis I SCID varied greatly by diagnosis and by site but generally fell somewhere among those reported for other diagnostic instruments, such as the National Institute of Mental Health Diagnostic Interview Schedule (DIS) (Robins et al. 1981), and the Schedule for Affective Disorders and Schizophrenia (SADS) (Endicott and Spitzer 1978). A number of newer studies using the SCID and focusing on particular diagnostic groups have reported much higher kappas, ranging from .70 to 1.00. These have used joint or videotaped interviews in determining reliability and therefore produce higher kappas because of the absence of information variance (Segal et al. 1993, 1994, 1995; Strakowski et al. 1993, 1995; Stukenberg et al. 1990).

The validity of a diagnostic assessment technique (procedural validity) refers to the agreement between the diagnoses made by the assessment technique and some hypothetical "gold standard." Unfortunately, a gold standard for psychiatric diagnosis remains elusive. There is obvious difficulty in using ordinary clinical diagnoses as the standard because structured interviews have been specifically designed to improve on the inherent limitations of an unstructured clinical interview. Spitzer has proposed a "LEAD" standard that could be used to evaluate the procedural validity of structured diagnostic interviews (Spitzer 1983). This standard involves longitudinal assessment (L), done by expert diagnosticians (E), using all data (AD) that are available about the subjects, such as family informants and the observations of clinical staff. Although conceptually the LEAD standard is appealing, the difficulty in implementing it accounts for its limited use. One study (Skodol et al. 1988) using the LEAD standard to evaluate structured diagnostic interviews compared the procedural validity of the SCID-II with an early version of the Personality Disorders Examination. The results indicated comparable but low agreement with the LEAD standard. A modification of the LEAD standard was used in the study by Basco et al. (unpublished) that investigated the utility of incorporating the SCID into the intake procedure of a community mental health center (discussed on page 1 of the User's Guide). In a study of substance abusers by Kranzler et al. (1995), diagnoses obtained using the SCID demonstrated superior validity when compared with the standard clinical interview on intake.

12. Data Processing

Unlike some other structured diagnostic interviews, the SCID-CV does not require the use of a computer program to make the final DSM-IV diagnoses. However, several relevant software packages are either currently available or in development from Multi-Health Systems of Toronto, Canada. More information is available by calling 1-(800)-456-3003.

1. SCID-SCREEN-PQ is a computer-administered, patient self-report, screening version of the SCID that presents the initial probe questions for the different modules of the SCID. It does *not* make diagnoses but instead produces a report indicating the diagnoses that are suggested (or unlikely) based on the patient's responses. It is currently available in both a DOS-compatible and Windows-compatible version.

2. A computer-administered version of the SCID-CV is being developed for a Windows environment. Call Multi-Health Systems regarding availability.

13. References

American Psychiatric Association: Diagnostic and Statistical Manual of Mental Disorders, Third Edition. Washington, DC, American Psychiatric Association, 1980

American Psychiatric Association: Diagnostic and Statistical Manual of Mental Disorders, Third Edition, Revised. Washington, DC, American Psychiatric Association, 1987

American Psychiatric Association: Diagnostic and Statistical Manual of Mental Disorders, Fourth Edition. Washington, DC, American Psychiatric Association, 1994

Endicott J, Spitzer RL: A diagnostic interview: the schedule for affective disorders and schizophrenia. Arch Gen Psychiatry 35: 837–844, 1978

Feighner JP, Robins E, Guze SB, et al: Diagnostic criteria for use in psychiatric research. Arch Gen Psychiatry 26:57–63, 1972

First MB, Spitzer RL, Gibbon M, et al: User's Guide for the Structured Clinical Interview for DSM-IV Personality Disorders (SCID-II).

Washington, DC, American Psychiatric Press, in press

Kranzler HR, Ronald MN, Burleson JA, et al: Validity of psychiatric diagnoses in patients with substance use disorders: is the interview more important than the interviewer? Compr Psychiatry 36:278–288, 1995

Robins LN, Helzer JE, Croughan J, et al: National Institute of Mental Health Diagnostic Interview Schedule: its history, characteristics, and validity. Arch Gen Psychiatry 38: 381–389, 1981

Segal DL, Hersen M, Van Hasselt VB, et al: Reliability of diagnosis in older psychiatric patients using the structured clinical interview for DSM-III-R. Journal of Psychopathology and Behavioral Assessment 15:347–356, 1993

Segal DL, Hersen M, Van Hasselt VB: Reliability of the Structured Clinical Interview for DSM-III-R: an evaluative review. Compr Psychiatry 35:316–327, 1994

Segal DL, Kabacoff RI, Hersen M, et al: Update on the reliability of diagnosis in older psychiatric outpatients using the Structured Clinical Interview for DSM-III-R. Journal of Clinical Geropsychology 1:313–321, 1995

Skodol AE, Rosnick L, Kellman D, et al: Validating structured DSM-III-R personality disorder assessments with longitudinal data. Am J Psychiatry 145:1297–1299, 1988

Spitzer RL: Psychiatric diagnosis: are clinicians still necessary? Compr Psychiatry 24: 399–411, 1983

Spitzer RL, Cohen J, Fleiss JL, et al: Quantification of agreement in psychiatric diagnosis: a new approach. Arch Gen Psychiatry 17: 83–87, 1967

Spitzer RL, Endicott J, Robins E: Research Diagnostic Criteria. Arch Gen Psychiatry 35: 773–782, 1978

Spitzer RL, Williams JBW, Gibbon M, et al: The Structured Clinical Interview for DSM-III-R (SCID), I: history, rationale, and description. Arch Gen Psychiatry 49:625–629, 1992

Spitzer RL, Gibbon M, Skodol AE, et al: DSM-IV Casebook. Washington, DC, American Psychiatric Press, 1994

Strakowski SM, Tohen M, Stoll AL, et al: Comorbidity in psychosis at first hospitalization. Am J Psychiatry 150:752–757, 1993

Strakowski SM, Keck PE, McElroy SL, et al: Chronology of comorbid and principal syndromes in first-episode psychosis. Compr Psychiatry 36:106–112, 1995

Stukenberg KW, Dura JR, Kiecolt-Glaser JK: Depression screening scale validation in an elderly, community-dwelling population. Psychological Assessment 2:134–138, 1990

Williams JBW, Gibbon M, First MB, et al: The Structured Clinical Interview for DSM-III-R (SCID), II: multi-site test-retest reliability. Arch Gen Psychiatry 49:630–636, 1992

14. Appendix: Training Materials

Two types of sample cases are included for training. The six *role-play cases* are useful for practicing how to administer the SCID-CV. These role-play cases work best in groups of two to four, with one person assuming the role of the SCID-CV interviewer, a second person assuming the role of the patient, and the remaining participants acting as observers, making ratings along with the interviewer. Each case should be read by the "patient" only—the other members of the group should remain unaware of the case so that the psychopathology can be revealed as the role-play develops. The "patient" should start by reading the Overview section aloud to the other members of the group. This is in lieu of doing the Overview, which we have found to be particularly difficult to role-play. The interviewer should begin the practice interview with the A module (page 3 in the Administration Booklet, page 13 in the Scoresheet). The person playing the patient should follow the instructions about how to answer the questions so that multiple small groups doing the role-play in parallel will arrive at the same diagnosis. After each role-play case, it is suggested that the entire group discuss the case together, focusing on any discrepancies among groups. Sample pages of the relevant SCID-CV modules demonstrating correct ratings are included for the following cases (following each case): Depressed Truck Driver, Weather Woman, Guy From the FBI, Drug Store, and Panic at the Airport. Sample pages are not included for Junior

Executive because it covers the same SCID sections as Depressed Truck Driver. For Depressed Truck Driver, we have included the Diagnostic Summary (Mood Disorders only), Overview, and Modules A and D. For Weather Woman, we have included the Diagnostic Summary (Mood Disorders only) and Modules A, B, C, and D. For Guy From the FBI, the Diagnostic Summary (Psychotic Disorders only) and Modules B and C. For Drug Store, the Diagnostic Summary (Substance Use Disorders only) and Module E. For Panic at the Airport, the Diagnostic Summary (Anxiety Disorders only) and Module F. Pages on which there are no ratings have not been included.

The next seven *homework cases* (from the *DSM-IV Casebook* [Spitzer et al. 1994][1], with a few changes in some cases to make it easier to apply the diagnostic criteria) are intended to help the clinician practice how to navigate through the C module of the SCID-CV. When administering the SCID-CV, the clinician is expected to go through the C module with the patient sitting in front of him or her so that the clinician has the opportunity to ask additional clarifying questions. It is therefore advisable for the clinician to become proficient in using the C module. Each case should be read and then "coded" as if one were administering the SCID-CV to that patient, starting at the beginning of the A module. If information for rating a particular criterion is not mentioned in the case example, assume that it has not been present and assign a rating of "–." The discussion following each case indicates the correct "pathway" through the SCID-CV, given the ratings in the case.

---

[1] From Spitzer RL, Gibbon M, Skodol AE, et al: *DSM-IV Casebook*. Washington, DC, American Psychiatric Press, 1994. Used with permission. Copyright 1994 American Psychiatric Press, Inc.

Role-Play—Case 1

"Depressed Truck Driver"

OVERVIEW: [Read this to the interviewer] This 60-year-old truck driver says he has been depressed for the past 6 months and has been unable to go to work. He also reports that he has been avoiding his friends and no longer likes to venture out of the house. He had a similar episode 10 years ago. Between these episodes he has felt well.

MOOD SYMPTOMS: Acknowledge persistent depression, loss of interest, 20-pound weight loss, insomnia, psychomotor retardation, and guilt, but do not give details unless the interviewer asks for them. If asked, give enough concrete information to substantiate that symptoms have been present most of the day, nearly every day for months. When asked about guilt, explain that your son has a drug problem, and you worry that it's because you were on the road so much and didn't spend time with him when he was a little boy. You are in good health and have not started using (nor increased the amount of) alcohol, drugs, or medications. This depression did not begin after someone close to you died.

Answer "no" to all other questions in the A module, except "yes" to the question about whether during the current month you have been shouting at people or starting fights or arguments—elaborate by reporting that all of the arguments have been confined to fighting with your wife about not wanting to go out of the house.

PSYCHOTIC AND ASSOCIATED SYMPTOMS: Answer "no" to everything except the first question about whether people pay special attention to you. In response to that, say that you stay inside because if you go on the street people keep asking why you're not at work. If asked for elaboration, make it clear that this is simple oversensitivity to the neighbors' vocal concerns and not a delusion of reference.

SUBSTANCE USE DISORDERS: You drink no more than two beers on an occasion, and that only rarely, and you have never used illegal drugs nor had any problem with prescribed drugs.

> *SCID Diagnosis:*
> Major Depressive Disorder, Recurrent, Severe, Without Psychotic Features
> *GAF:* 35
> (major impairment in several areas)

STRUCTURED CLINICAL INTERVIEW FOR DSM-IV AXIS I DISORDERS

SCID-I

CLINICIAN VERSION

SCORESHEET

Michael B. First, M.D.
Robert L. Spitzer, M.D.
Miriam Gibbon, M.S.W.
Janet B. W. Williams, D.S.W.

Biometrics Research Department
New York State Psychiatric Institute
Department of Psychiatry
Columbia University
New York, New York

Patient's name: _Depressed Truck Driver_

Record number: _005_   Date of evaluation: _1/29/96_

Clinician: _Gibbon_

Sources of information (check all that apply):
- ☒ Patient
- ❑ Family/friends/associates
- ❑ Health professional
- ☒ Medical records

SCID-CV DIAGNOSTIC SUMMARY

MOOD DISORDERS

Current Lifetime

Bipolar I Disorder (*D4,* p. 36)

☐ ☐ 296.40　Bipolar I Disorder, Most Recent Episode Hypomanic

☐ ☐ 296.0x　Bipolar I Disorder, Single Manic Episode

☐ ☐ 296.4x　Bipolar I Disorder, Most Recent Episode Manic

☐ ☐ 296.6x　Bipolar I Disorder, Most Recent Episode Mixed

☐ ☐ 296.5x　Bipolar I Disorder, Most Recent Episode Depressed
　　　　check fifth-digit specifier:
　　　　__ 1—Mild
　　　　__ 2—Moderate
　　　　__ 3—Severe, Without Psychotic Features
　　　　__ 4—Severe, With Psychotic Features
　　　　__ 5—In Partial Remission
　　　　__ 6—In Full Remission
　　　　__ 0—Unspecified

☐ ☐ 296.7　Bipolar I Disorder, Most Recent Episode Unspecified

Other Bipolar Disorders

☐ ☐ 296.89　Bipolar II Disorder (*D9,* p. 37)
　　　　check specifier:
　　　　___ Hypomanic
　　　　___ Depressed

☐ ☐ 301.13　Cyclothymic Disorder (*D12,* p. 37)

☐ ☐ 296.80　Bipolar Disorder Not Otherwise Specified (*D12,* p. 37)

Major Depressive Disorder (*D16,* p. 38)

☐ ☐ 296.2x　Major Depressive Disorder, Single Episode

☒ ☒ 296.3x　Major Depressive Disorder, Recurrent
　　　　check fifth-digit specifier:
　　　　__ 1—Mild
　　　　__ 2—Moderate
　　　　☒ 3—Severe, Without Psychotic Features
　　　　__ 4—Severe, With Psychotic Features
　　　　__ 5—In Partial Remission
　　　　__ 6—In Full Remission
　　　　__ 0—Unspecified

Other Depressive Disorders

☐ 　　300.4　Dysthymic Disorder (*A60,* p. 23)

☐ ☐ 311　　Depressive Disorder Not Otherwise Specified (*D19,* p. 39)

DSM-IV Axis V: Global Assessment of Functioning Scale

Consider psychological, social, and occupational functioning on a hypothetical continuum of mental health–illness. Do not include impairment in functioning as a result of physical (or environmental) limitations.

> **GAF rating:**
> current: **3 5**
> **highest past**
> **year:** **0 0 0**

CODE (**Note:** Use intermediate codes when appropriate, e.g., 45, 68, 72)

100   **Superior functioning in a wide range of activities, life's problems never seem to get out of hand, is sought out by others because of his or her many positive qualities. No symptoms.**
91

90   **Absent or minimal symptoms** (e.g., mild anxiety before an exam); **good functioning in all areas, interested and involved in a wide range of activities, socially effective, generally satisfied with life, no more than everyday problems or concerns** (e.g., an occasional argument with family
81   members).

80   **If symptoms are present, they are transient and expectable reactions to psychosocial stressors** (e.g., difficulty concentrating after family argument); **no more than slight impairment in**
71   **social, occupational, or school functioning** (e.g., temporarily falling behind in schoolwork).

70   **Some mild symptoms** (e.g., depressed mood and mild insomnia) **OR some difficulty in social, occupational, or school functioning** (e.g., occasional truancy, or theft within the household), **but**
61   **generally functioning pretty well, has some meaningful interpersonal relationships.**

60   **Moderate symptoms** (e.g., flat affect and circumstantial speech, occasional panic attacks) **OR**
51   **moderate difficulty in social, occupational, or school functioning** (e.g., few friends, conflicts with peers or co-workers).

50   **Serious symptoms** (e.g., suicidal ideation, severe obsessional rituals, frequent shoplifting) **OR any serious impairment in social, occupational, or school functioning** (e.g., no friends, unable to keep
41   a job).

40   **Some impairment in reality testing or communication** (e.g., speech is at times illogical, obscure, or irrelevant) **OR major impairment in several areas, such as work or school, family relations, judgment, thinking, or mood** (e.g., depressed man avoids friends, neglects family, and is unable to
31   work; child frequently beats up younger children, is defiant at home, and is failing at school).

30   **Behavior is considerably influenced by delusions or hallucinations OR serious impairment in communication or judgment** (e.g., sometimes incoherent, acts grossly inappropriately, suicidal
21   preoccupation) **OR inability to function in almost all areas** (e.g., stays in bed all day; no job, home, or friends).

20   **Some danger of hurting self or others** (e.g., suicide attempts without clear expectation of death, frequently violent, manic excitement) **OR occasionally fails to maintain minimal personal hygiene**
11   (e.g., smears feces) **OR gross impairment in communication** (e.g., largely incoherent or mute).

10   **Persistent danger of severely hurting self or others** (e.g., recurrent violence) **OR persistent inability to maintain minimal personal hygiene OR serious suicidal act with clear expectation**
1   **of death.**

0   Inadequate information.

OVERVIEW

DEMOGRAPHIC DATA

What's your date of birth?	*Date of Birth:* **7** **7** **35** month day year	**P1**
Are you married? IF NO: Were you ever?	*Marital Status:* ①—Married or living with someone as if married 2—Widowed 3—Divorced or annulled 3—Separated 4—Never married	**P2**
Any children? IF YES: How many?	2 (adult)	**P3**
Where do you live? Whom do you live with?	Forest Hills wife	**P4**

EDUCATIONAL HISTORY

How far did you get in school? IF FAILED TO COMPLETE A PROGRAM IN WHICH HE/SHE WAS ENROLLED: Why didn't you finish?	*Education:* 1—Grade 6 or less 2—Grade 7 to 12 (without graduating high school) ③—Graduated high school or high school equivalent 4—Part college 5—Graduated 2-year college/technical school 6—Graduated 4-year college 7—Part graduate/professional school 8—Completed graduate/professional school	**P5**

OCCUPATIONAL HISTORY

What kind of work do you do?
 	
Are you working now?
 	
┌IF YES: How long have you worked there?
 	
   IF LESS THAN 6 MONTHS: Why did you leave your last job?
 	
  Have you always done that kind of work?
 	
└IF NO: Why is that?
 	
What kind of work have you done before?
 	
How are you supporting yourself now?
	Truck driver
	Out of work 6 months—too depressed
	
	Worked for same company for 20 years
	
	Sick leave, disability
		P6

IF UNKNOWN: Has there ever been a period of time when you were unable to work or go to school? IF YES: When? Why was that?		**P7**

STATUS OF CURRENT TREATMENT

IF UNKNOWN: Have you been in any kind of treatment in the past month?	*Treatment Setting:* (Circle one) 1—Current inpatient (including residential treatment) ②—Current outpatient 3—Other (e.g., 12-step program such as AA) 4—No current treatment	**P8**
IF INPATIENT: When did you come into the hospital? IF OUTPATIENT: When did you start coming to the (clinic/office/program)?	*Date:* *1/29/96*	**P9**

CHIEF COMPLAINT AND DESCRIPTION OF PROBLEM

| What led to your coming here (this time)? (What is the major problem you are having trouble with?)

IF DOES NOT GIVE DETAILS OF PRESENTING PROBLEM: Tell me more about that. (What do you mean by... ?) | depressed, Can't work, not getting better

Wife insisted he get treatment— can't get out of house in the morning— doesn't want to do anything. | P10 |

ONSET OF PRESENT ILLNESS OR EXACERBATION

| When did this begin? (When did you first notice that something was wrong?)

When were you last feeling OK (your usual self)? | July 1995 — hard to get up & get to work, very tired | P11 |

NEW SYMPTOMS OR RECURRENCE

| Is this something new or a return of something you had before?

(What made you come for help now?) | similar episode 10 years ago

wife | P12 |

ENVIRONMENTAL CONTEXT AND POSSIBLE PRECIPITANTS (USE FOR REPORTING AXIS IV)

| Did anything happen or change just before this all started?

(Do you think this had anything to do with your [PRESENT ILLNESS])?

What other kinds of problems were you having when this began? | Nothing special | P13 |

COURSE OF PRESENT ILLNESS OR EXACERBATION

After it started, what happened next? (Did other things start to bother you?)	lost appetite, couldn't sleep. no energy to go to work.	P14
Since this began, when have you felt the worst? IF MORE THAN A YEAR AGO: In the last year, when have you felt the worst?	Now	P15

TREATMENT HISTORY

When was the first time you saw someone for emotional or psychiatric problems? (What was that for? What treatment(s) did you get? What medications?) What about treatment for drugs or alcohol? (THE LIFE CHART ON PAGE 12 OF THE SCORESHEET MAY BE USED TO DOCUMENT A COMPLICATED HISTORY OF PSYCHOPATHOLOGY AND TREATMENT)	1985— depressed Tofranil— better in a few months— stopped going to clinic None	P16
Have you ever been a patient in a psychiatric hospital? IF YES: What was that for? (How many times?) IF GIVES AN INADEQUATE ANSWER, CHALLENGE GENTLY: e.g., Wasn't there something else? People don't usually go to psychiatric hospitals just because they are [TIRED/ NERVOUS/OWN WORDS].	No prior hospitalization	P17
Have you ever been a patient in a hospital for treatment of a medical problem? IF YES: What was that for?	Hernia repair, 1990	P18

OTHER CURRENT PROBLEMS

Have you had any other problems in the past month?	*No*	**P19**
What has your mood been like?	*Depressed*	**P20**
How has you physical health been? (Have you had any medical problems?) (USE THIS INFORMATION TO REPORT AXIS III)	*OK*	**P21**
Do you take any medications or vitamins (other than those you have already told me about)? IF YES: How much and how often do you take [MEDICATION]? (Has there been any change in the amount you have been taking?)	*None*	**P22**
How much have you been drinking [alcohol] [in the past month]? Have you been taking any drugs [in the past month]? (What about marijuana, cocaine, other street drugs?)	*Nothing now*	**P23**

CURRENT SOCIAL FUNCTIONING (USE FOR REPORTING AXIS V)

How have you been spending your free time?	*Watching TV, trying to sleep*	**P24**
Whom do you spend time with?	*Wife*	

OVERVIEW DIAGNOSES

MOST LIKELY CURRENT DIAGNOSIS: *Major Depressive Disorder*	P25
DIAGNOSES THAT NEED TO BE RULED OUT:	P26

LIFE CHART

Age (or date)	Description (symptoms, triggering events)	Treatment
_____	_____	_____
_____	_____	_____
_____	_____	_____
_____	_____	_____
_____	_____	_____
_____	_____	_____
_____	_____	_____
_____	_____	_____
_____	_____	_____
_____	_____	_____
_____	_____	_____
_____	_____	_____
_____	_____	_____
_____	_____	_____
_____	_____	_____
_____	_____	_____

A. MOOD EPISODES

MAJOR DEPRESSIVE EPISODE CRITERIA

onset of episode: ____

check if: current   ✓
        past   ____
if past, offset: ____

A. Five (or more) . . . during the same 2 weeks . . . at least one of the symptoms is either (1) depressed mood, or (2) loss of interest or pleasure.

A1

(1) depressed mood
Notes:

            ?   −   ⊕   **A1**

A2

(2) markedly diminished interest or pleasure
Notes: No interest in work, sports, seeing friends—doesn't want to do anything

            ?   −   ⊕   **A2**
                A16 p. 15

A3

(3) weight loss/gain; decreased/increased appetite
Notes: 20-lb weight loss

            ?   −   ⊕   **A3**

A4

(4) insomnia or hypersomnia
Notes: Can't get to sleep for hours

            ?   −   ⊕   **A4**

A5

(5) psychomotor agitation or retardation
Notes: apparent during interview

            ?   −   ⊕   **A5**

Ratings: ? = Inadequate information;   − = Absent (or subthreshold);   + = Present

A6	(6) fatigue or loss of energy *Notes:* no energy	? − ⊕
A7	(7) feelings of worthlessness or (excessive or inappropriate guilt) *Notes:* unreasonably takes responsibility for son's longstanding drug problem	? − ⊕
A8	(8) diminished ability to think or indecisiveness *Notes:*	? ⊖ +
A9	(9) thoughts of death, suicidal ideation, attempt, or plan *Notes:*	? ⊖ +
A10	**AT LEAST FIVE OF A(1)–A(9) ARE "+" AND AT LEAST ONE OF THESE IS A(1) OR A(2)**	? − ⊕ A16 p. 15
A11	C. Clinically significant impairment or distress *Notes:* Can't work	? − ⊕ A16 p. 15
A12	D. Not due to a substance or a general medical condition (check p. 24) *WARNING: A "YES" answer to the interview question equals a "−" rating* *Notes:*	? − ⊕ A16 p. 15

Ratings: ? = Inadequate information;   − = Absent (or subthreshold);   + = Present

| A13 | E. Not better accounted for by Bereavement
WARNING: A "YES" answer to the interview question equals a "–" rating | ? ⊤ ⊕
A16
p. 15 | A13 |

| A14 | **CRITERIA A, C, D, AND E ARE "+"**

Check here ✓ if criteria have been met in the past month. | ⊕
↓
Major Depressive Episode | A14 |

| A15 | Total number of Major Depressive Episodes | 0 2 | A15 |

MANIC EPISODE CRITERIA

onset of episode: ____

check if: current ____
             past ____
if past, offset: ____

| A16 | A. Abnormally and persistently elevated, expansive, or irritable mood . . .
Notes: | ? ⊖ +
A45
p. 21 | A16 |

| A17 | . . . lasting at least 1 week (or any duration if hospitalization is necessary)
Notes: | ? ⊤ +
A30
p. 18 | A17 |

| | B. During the period of mood disturbance, three (or more) of the following symptoms have persisted (four if the mood is only irritable) and have been present to a significant degree: | | |

| A18 | (1) inflated self-esteem or grandiosity
Notes: | ? – + | A18 |

Ratings: ? = Inadequate information;   – = Absent (or subthreshold);   + = Present

DYSTHYMIC DISORDER CRITERIA

A45	A. Depressed mood for most of the day, for more days than not for at least 2 years *Notes:*	? ⊖ + **B1** p. 26	A45
	B. Presence of two (or more) of the following:		
A46	(1) poor appetite or overeating *Notes:*	? — +	A46
A47	(2) insomnia or hypersomnia *Notes:*	? — +	A47
A48	(3) low energy or fatigue *Notes:*	? — +	A48
A49	(4) low self-esteem *Notes:*	? — +	A49
A50	(5) poor concentration or difficulty making decisions *Notes:*	? — +	A50

Ratings: ? = Inadequate information; – = Absent (or subthreshold); + = Present

D. MOOD DISORDERS

BIPOLAR I DISORDER CRITERIA

E1
p. 40

D1	History of one or more Manic or Mixed Episodes (see **A28**, p. 17)	(no) yes D5 p. 37	**D1**
D2	At least one Manic or Mixed Episode is not due to a general medical condition or substance use.	no yes D5 p. 37	**D2**
D3	At least one Manic or Mixed Episode is not better accounted for by Schizoaffective Disorder and is not superimposed on Schizophrenia, Schizophreniform Disorder, Delusional Disorder, or Psychotic Disorder Not Otherwise Specified.	no yes D5 p. 37	**D3**

D4	BIPOLAR I DISORDER: Select first four digits of diagnostic code based on current (or most recent) episode (fifth digit indicates severity).		**D4**

E1
p. 40

Check here ___ if criteria have been met in the past month.

Check one:
___ **296.40 Most Recent Episode Hypomanic**

___ **296.0x Single Manic Episode**
___ **296.4x Most Recent Episode Manic**
___ **296.6x Most Recent Episode Mixed**
___ **296.5x Most Recent Episode Depressed**

Check fifth digit:
__ 1—Mild
__ 2—Moderate
__ 3—Severe, Without Psychotic Features
__ 4—Severe, With Psychotic Features
__ 5—In Partial Remission
__ 6—In Full Remission
__ 0—Unspecified

___ **296.7 Most Recent Episode Unspecified**

BIPOLAR II DISORDER CRITERIA

D5	At least one Hypomanic Episode not due to a general medical condition or substance use (see **A43**, p. 20)	(no) yes → **D10** below	D5
D6	At least one Major Depressive Episode not due to a general medical condition or substance use (see **A14**, p. 15)	no yes → **D10** below	D6
D7	Never any Manic or Mixed Episodes	no yes → **D10** below	D7
D8	Not better accounted for by Schizoaffective Disorder and not superimposed on Schizophrenia, Schizophreniform Disorder, Delusional Disorder, or Psychotic Disorder Not Otherwise Specified	no yes → **D10** below	D8
D9	Check one based on current (or most recent) episode: __ **296.89 Bipolar II Disorder, Hypomanic** __ **296.89 Bipolar II Disorder, Depressed** Check here ___ if criteria have been met in the past month.	**E1** p. 40	D9

OTHER BIPOLAR DISORDERS

D10	Clinically significant manic or hypomanic symptoms	(no) yes → **D13** p. 38	D10
D11	Not due to a substance or a general medical condition (check p. 24)	no yes → **D13** p. 38	D11
D12	Indicate type: __ **301.13 Cyclothymic Disorder** __ **296.80 Bipolar Disorder Not Otherwise Specified** Check here ___ if present in past month.	**E1** p. 40	D12

Ratings: ? = Inadequate information;   – = Absent (or subthreshold);   + = Present

MAJOR DEPRESSIVE DISORDER CRITERIA

D13   At least one Major Depressive Episode that is not due to a general medical condition or substance use (see **A14**, p. 15)   **no**   (**yes**)   **D13**

D17 p. 39

D14   Not better accounted for by Schizoaffective Disorder and not superimposed on Schizophrenia, Schizophreniform Disorder, Delusional Disorder, or Psychotic Disorder Not Otherwise Specified   **no**   (**yes**)   **D14**

D17 p. 39

D15   Never any Manic, Mixed, or Hypomanic Episodes   **no**   (**yes**)   **D15**

D17 p. 39

D16   **MAJOR DEPRESSIVE DISORDER** Select first four digits based on number of episodes (fifth digit indicates severity)   E1 p. 40   **D16**

Check here ✓ if criteria have been met in the past month.

Check one:
___ **296.2x Major Depressive Disorder, Single Episode**
✗ **296.3x Major Depressive Disorder, Recurrent**

Check fifth digit:
___ 1—Mild
___ 2—Moderate
✗ 3—Severe, Without Psychotic Features
___ 4—Severe, With Psychotic Features
___ 5—In Partial Remission
___ 6—In Full Remission
___ 0—Unspecified

DEPRESSIVE DISORDER NOT OTHERWISE SPECIFIED

D17	Clinically significant depressive symptoms	**no** **yes**	D17
		E1 p. 40	
D18	Not due to a substance or a general medical condition (check p. 24)	**no** **yes**	D18
		E1 p. 40	
D19	**311 Depressive Disorder Not Otherwise Specified** Check here ___ if present in the past month.	E1 p. 40	D19

Ratings: ? = Inadequate information; – = Absent (or subthreshold); + = Present

Role-Play—Case 2

"The Weather Woman"

OVERVIEW: [Read this to the interviewer] A 50-year-old woman is brought to the hospital by her family because she has not been sleeping and her behavior has been increasingly bizarre over the past 3 weeks. She is very angry about her hospitalization, believing that her family just wants to prevent her from getting her good news to the world.

MOOD SYMPTOMS: Answer "never" to all questions about depression and loss of interest. In response to the question about elevated mood, explain that you are feeling "joyous" about your newly discovered ability to control the weather. About "special powers" (criterion B[1]), explain that you have been granted the ability to control the weather and thereby end drought, disperse smog, reverse the greenhouse effect, and turn the world into Eden.

About your sleeping (criterion B[2]), say that you have not slept for 10 days because you are so excited about your new powers. About talking too much (criterion B[3]), either demonstrate over-talkativeness, or tell the interviewer that your family is complaining that you talk too much. In response to the question about racing thoughts (criterion B[4]), say your mind is "flooded" with ideas about your new project. In answer to distractibility (criterion B[5]), say "yes," but don't give any examples. About increase in activities (criterion B[6]), say you have been going all over town to television and radio stations to try to get the news out. About doing anything that could get you in trouble (criterion B[7]), say that you got arrested when you tried to get in to see Mike Wallace.

You are and have always been in excellent health and you deny having any alcohol or drugs of any kind for the past several years.

PSYCHOTIC AND ASSOCIATED SYMPTOMS: Answer "no" to people talking about you or taking special notice of you. In response to receiving special messages from the television, explain that it is your message you have been trying to get to the television people.

About persecutory delusions, say your family thinks you are crazy because they fail to understand the importance of your new powers, and you are angry at them for railroading you into the hospital. In response to questions about grandiose delusions, explain how you have had this revelation from "the deities" about how to control the weather. Answer "no" to all other specific questions about delusions.

In response to questions about whether you hear voices, explain that these "deities" are not really voices, but you awoke one morning with the knowledge about how to control the weather and then understood that it had come from "the deities." In fact, you do not hear actual voices at all. Say "no" to all other hallucinations.

SUBSTANCE USE DISORDERS: You report having tried marijuana once and did not like it and that you have never liked alcohol.

SCID Diagnosis:
  Bipolar I Disorder, Manic, Severe With
  Psychotic Features
GAF: 21
  (behavior is considerably influenced by
  delusions and has gotten her into trouble)

SCID - I

CLINICIAN VERSION

SCORESHEET

Michael B. First, M.D.
Robert L. Spitzer, M.D.
Miriam Gibbon, M.S.W.
Janet B. W. Williams, D.S.W.

Biometrics Research Department
New York State Psychiatric Institute
Department of Psychiatry
Columbia University
New York, New York

Patient's name: _Weather Woman_

Record number: _014_   Date of evaluation: _10/8/91_

Clinician: _First_

Sources of information (check all that apply):   ☒ Patient

   ☐ Family/friends/associates

   ☐ Health professional

   ☐ Medical records

SCID-CV DIAGNOSTIC SUMMARY

MOOD DISORDERS

Current	Lifetime	
		Bipolar I Disorder (*D4*, p. 36)
☐	☐	296.40 Bipolar I Disorder, Most Recent Episode Hypomanic
☒	☒	296.0x Bipolar I Disorder, Single Manic Episode
☐	☐	296.4x Bipolar I Disorder, Most Recent Episode Manic
☐	☐	296.6x Bipolar I Disorder, Most Recent Episode Mixed
☐	☐	296.5x Bipolar I Disorder, Most Recent Episode Depressed

check fifth-digit specifier:
__ 1—Mild
__ 2—Moderate
__ 3—Severe, Without Psychotic Features
✗ 4—Severe, With Psychotic Features
__ 5—In Partial Remission
__ 6—In Full Remission
__ 0—Unspecified

Current	Lifetime	
☐	☐	296.7 Bipolar I Disorder, Most Recent Episode Unspecified

Other Bipolar Disorders

Current	Lifetime	
☐	☐	296.89 Bipolar II Disorder (*D9*, p. 37)

check specifier:
___ Hypomanic
___ Depressed

Current	Lifetime	
☐	☐	301.13 Cyclothymic Disorder (*D12*, p. 37)
☐	☐	296.80 Bipolar Disorder Not Otherwise Specified (*D12*, p. 37)

Major Depressive Disorder (*D16*, p. 38)

Current	Lifetime	
☐	☐	296.2x Major Depressive Disorder, Single Episode
☐	☐	296.3x Major Depressive Disorder, Recurrent

check fifth-digit specifier:
__ 1—Mild
__ 2—Moderate
__ 3—Severe, Without Psychotic Features
__ 4—Severe, With Psychotic Features
__ 5—In Partial Remission
__ 6—In Full Remission
__ 0—Unspecified

Other Depressive Disorders

Current	Lifetime	
☐		300.4 Dysthymic Disorder (*A60*, p. 23)
☐	☐	311 Depressive Disorder Not Otherwise Specified (*D19*, p. 39)

A13	E. Not better accounted for by Bereavement *WARNING: A "YES" answer to the interview question equals a "–" rating*	? ─ + **A16** p. 15	**A13**
A14	**CRITERIA A, C, D, AND E ARE "+"** Check here ___ if criteria have been met in the past month.	+ ↓ **Major Depressive Episode**	**A14**
A15	Total number of Major Depressive Episodes	＿＿	**A15**

MANIC EPISODE CRITERIA

onset of episode: ＿＿

check if: current ✓
         past ＿＿
   if past, offset: ＿＿

A16	A. Abnormally and persistently elevated, expansive, or irritable mood . . . *Notes:* feeling "joyous"	? ─ ⊕ **A45** p. 21	**A16**
A17	. . . lasting at least 1 week (or any duration if (hospitalization) is necessary) *Notes:*	? ─ ⊕ **A30** p. 18	**A17**
	B. During the period of mood disturbance, three (or more) of the following symptoms have persisted (four if the mood is only irritable) and have been present to a significant degree:		
A18	(1) inflated self-esteem or grandiosity *Notes:* Controlling the weather	? ─ ⊕	**A18**

Ratings: ? = Inadequate information;   – = Absent (or subthreshold);   + = Present

A19	(2) decreased need for sleep *Notes:* no sleep for 10 days	?　　–　　⊕　　**A19**
A20	(3) more talkative than usual or pressured speech *Notes:* talks very fast — hard to 　　　interrupt	?　　–　　⊕　　**A20**
A21	(4) flight of ideas or racing thoughts *Notes:* mind "flooded" with ideas	?　　–　　⊕　　**A21**
A22	(5) distractibility *Notes:*	?　　⊖　　+　　**A22**
A23	(6) increase in goal-directed activity or psychomotor agitation *Notes:* running around to TV & 　radio stations	?　　–　　⊕　　**A23**
A24	(7) excessive involvement in pleasurable activities *Notes:* not for pleasure, 2° to delusion	?　　⊖　　+　　**A24**
A25	**AT LEAST THREE OF B(1)–B(7) ARE "+" (OR FOUR IF MOOD IS IRRITABLE AND NOT ELEVATED)**	?　　–　　⊕　　**A25** ┌─────┐ │ A45 │ │ p. 21 │ └─────┘

Ratings:　? = Inadequate information;　　– = Absent (or subthreshold);　　+ = Present

A26	D. Sufficiently severe to cause marked impairment *Notes:* family insisted on hospitalization because of bizarre behavior	? − ⊕ A39 p. 19	A26
A27	E. Not due to a substance or a general medical condition (check p. 24) *WARNING: A "YES" answer to the interview question equals a "−" rating* *Notes:*	? − ⊕ A45 p. 21	A27
A28	**CRITERIA A, C, D, AND E ARE "+"** Check here ✔ if criteria have been met in the past month.	⊕ ↓ **Manic Episode**	A28
A29	Total number of Manic Episodes	0 1 B1 p. 26	A29

Ratings: ? = Inadequate information;   − = Absent (or subthreshold);   + = Present

B. PSYCHOTIC AND ASSOCIATED SYMPTOMS

B1	Delusion of reference *Describe:*	? ⊖ + **B1**
B2	Persecutory delusion *Describe:*	? ⊖ + **B2**
B3	Grandiose delusion *Describe:* Controlling the weather	? − ⊕ **B3**
B4	Somatic delusion *Describe:*	? ⊖ + **B4**
B5	Other delusions *Describe:*	? ⊖ + **B5**
B6	Auditory hallucinations *Describe:*	? ⊖ + **B6**
B7	Visual hallucinations *Describe:*	? ⊖ + **B7**

Ratings: ? = Inadequate information;   − = Absent (or subthreshold);   + = Present

B8	Tactile hallucinations *Describe:*	? (−) + **B8**
B9	Other hallucinations *Describe:*	? (−) + **B9**
B10	Catatonic behaviors *Describe:*	? (−) + **B10**
B11	Grossly disorganized behavior *Describe:*	? (−) + **B11**
B12	Grossly inappropriate affect *Describe:*	? (−) + **B12**
B13	Disorganized speech *Describe:*	? (−) + **B13**
B14	Negative symptoms *Describe:*	? (−) + **B14**

Ratings: ? = Inadequate information;   − = Absent (or subthreshold);   + = Present

C. DIFFERENTIAL DIAGNOSIS OF PSYCHOTIC DISORDERS

D1
p. 36

| C1 | Psychotic symptoms occur at times other than during mood episodes | (no)   **yes**
 D1 p. 36 | C1 |

SCHIZOPHRENIA CRITERIA

C2	A. One month of active-phase symptoms	**no** **yes** **C21** p. 32	C2
C3	D. Schizoaffective Disorder and Mood Disorder With Psychotic Features have been ruled out	**no** **yes** **C16** p. 31	C3
C4	C. Duration of 6 months	**no** **yes** **C13** p. 30	C4
C5	B. Functioning markedly impaired	**no** **yes** **C39** p. 35	C5
C6	E. Not due to a substance or a general medical condition (check p. 34)	**no** **yes** **D1** p. 36	C6
C7	**CRITERIA A, B, C, D, AND E ARE MET** Check here ___ if criteria have been met in the past month	**Schizophrenia**	C7

D. MOOD DISORDERS

BIPOLAR I DISORDER CRITERIA

E1
p. 40

| D1 | History of one or more Manic or Mixed Episodes (see **A28,** p. 17) | no   (yes) | D1 |
| | | D5
p. 37 | |

| D2 | At least one Manic or Mixed Episode is not due to a general medical condition or substance use. | no   (yes) | D2 |
| | | D5
p. 37 | |

| D3 | At least one Manic or Mixed Episode is not better accounted for by Schizoaffective Disorder and is not superimposed on Schizophrenia, Schizophreniform Disorder, Delusional Disorder, or Psychotic Disorder Not Otherwise Specified. | no   (yes) | D3 |
| | | D5
p. 37 | |

D4

BIPOLAR I DISORDER: Select first four digits of diagnostic code based on current (or most recent) episode (fifth digit indicates severity).

Check here ✓ if criteria have been met in the past month.

Check one:
___ **296.40 Most Recent Episode Hypomanic**

X 296.0x Single Manic Episode
___ **296.4x Most Recent Episode Manic**
___ **296.6x Most Recent Episode Mixed**
___ **296.5x Most Recent Episode Depressed**

Check fifth digit:
__ 1—Mild
__ 2—Moderate
__ 3—Severe, Without Psychotic Features
X 4—Severe, With Psychotic Features
__ 5—In Partial Remission
__ 6—In Full Remission
__ 0—Unspecified

___ **296.7 Most Recent Episode Unspecified**

D4

E1
p. 40

Role-Play—Case 3

"Guy From the FBI"

OVERVIEW: [Read this to the interviewer] This is a 35-year-old female secretary who says she has been "pursued" by a federal agent ever since she appeared in court for a speeding ticket 10 years ago.

MOOD SYMPTOMS: In response to question about depression, say your mood is "distraught" and "upset," and you have felt that way for weeks. Answer "no" to all the depressive symptom questions except for having trouble falling asleep, and trouble concentrating, because you are so frightened about what the FBI agent means to do to you.

Answer "no" to all manic questions. In response to the initial question for Dysthymic Disorder (page 17 of the Administration Booklet), say that, although the court appearance occurred 10 years ago, it is only in the past few weeks that you have realized he is stalking you and have been so upset. Therefore, you have not been depressed more days than not in the past 2 years.

PSYCHOTIC AND ASSOCIATED SYMPTOMS: In response to the initial question, explain that he is the only one who is paying special attention to you. You know this because you see him hanging around outside your building at night. Also say you get hang-ups on your answering machine that you are sure are from him. In response to the question about persecutory delusions, say you are not sure what he wants from you, but you think it is something sexual.

Answer "no" to all other delusions.

Answer "no" to all hallucinations. If the interviewer pushes about visual hallucinations, explain that you have seen him night after night, hanging around your street, dressed in a beige raincoat and a baseball cap. He is not close enough to see his features, but you are sure it is him.

You have no medical problems and deny any drug or alcohol use and you are not taking any medications.

> *SCID Diagnosis:*
>   Delusional Disorder
> *GAF:* 29
>   (behavior is influenced by delusions but less so than in previous case)

S C I D - I

CLINICIAN VERSION

SCORESHEET

Michael B. First, M.D.
Robert L. Spitzer, M.D.
Miriam Gibbon, M.S.W.
Janet B. W. Williams, D.S.W.

Biometrics Research Department
New York State Psychiatric Institute
Department of Psychiatry
Columbia University
New York, New York

Patient's name: _Guy From the FBI_

Record number: _666_ Date of evaluation: _2/1/96_

Clinician: _First_

Sources of information (check all that apply):
- ☒ Patient
- ☐ Family/friends/associates
- ☒ Health professional
- ☐ Medical records

Current Lifetime   **Other Mood Disorders**

❏   ❏   293.83   Mood Disorder Due to General Medical Condition (*A64*, p. 24)

Indicate General Medical Condition: _____

check specifier:
___ Major Depressive–like Episode
___ Other Depressive Symptoms
___ Manic
___ Mixed

❏   ❏   291.8   Alcohol-Induced Mood Disorder (*A69*, p. 25)

check specifier:
___ Depressed
___ Manic
___ Mixed

❏   ❏   292.84   Other Substance-Induced Mood Disorder *(A69*, p. 25)

Indicate substance: _____

check specifier:
___ Depressed
___ Manic
___ Mixed

SCHIZOPHRENIA AND OTHER PSYCHOTIC DISORDERS

❏   ❏   Schizophrenia (*C7*, p. 29)

check specifier:
___ 295.30 Paranoid Type (*C8*, p. 30)
___ 295.20 Catatonic Type (*C9*, p. 30)
___ 295.10 Disorganized Type (*C10*, p. 30)
___ 295.90 Undifferentiated Type (*C11*, p. 30)
___ 295.60 Residual Type (*C12*, p. 30)

❏   ❏   295.40   Schizophreniform Disorder (*C15*, p. 30)

❏   ❏   295.70   Schizoaffective Disorder (*C20*, p. 31)

☒   ☒   297.1   Delusional Disorder (*C26*, p. 32)

❏   ❏   298.8   Brief Psychotic Disorder (*C31*, p. 33)

❏   ❏   293.81   Psychotic Disorder Due to a General Medical Condition With Delusions (*C34*, p. 34)

Indicate General Medical Condition: _____

❏   ❏   293.82   Psychotic Disorder Due to a General Medical Condition With Hallucinations (*C34*, p. 34)

Indicate General Medical Condition: _____

❏   ❏   291.5   Alcohol-Induced Psychotic Disorder With Delusions (*C38*, p. 35)

❏   ❏   291.3   Alcohol-Induced Psychotic Disorder With Hallucinations (*C38*, p. 35)

❏   ❏   292.11   Other Substance-Induced Psychotic Disorder With Delusions (*C38*, p. 35)

Indicate substance: _____

❏   ❏   292.12   Other Substance-Induced Psychotic Disorder With Hallucinations (*C38*, p. 35)

Indicate substance: _____

❏   ❏   298.9   Psychotic Disorder Not Otherwise Specified (*C39*, p. 35)

B. PSYCHOTIC AND ASSOCIATED SYMPTOMS

B1	Delusion of reference *Describe:* FBI guy hanging around in street; phone hang ups	? − (+)	**B1**
B2	Persecutory delusion *Describe:* FBI guy stalking her	? − (+)	**B2**
B3	Grandiose delusion *Describe:*	? (−) +	**B3**
B4	Somatic delusion *Describe:*	? (−) +	**B4**
B5	Other delusions *Describe:*	? (−) +	**B5**
B6	Auditory hallucinations *Describe:*	? (−) +	**B6**
B7	Visual hallucinations *Describe:*	? (−) +	**B7**

Ratings: ? = Inadequate information;   − = Absent (or subthreshold);   + = Present

B8	Tactile hallucinations *Describe:*	? ⊖ +	B8
B9	Other hallucinations *Describe:*	? ⊖ +	B9
B10	Catatonic behaviors *Describe:*	? ⊖ +	B10
B11	Grossly disorganized behavior *Describe:*	? ⊖ +	B11
B12	Grossly inappropriate affect *Describe:*	? ⊖ +	B12
B13	Disorganized speech *Describe:*	? ⊖ +	B13
B14	Negative symptoms *Describe:*	? ⊖ +	B14

Ratings: ? = Inadequate information; − = Absent (or subthreshold); + = Present

B15

CHRONOLOGY OF PSYCHOTIC SYMPTOMS

B15

If any delusions or hallucinations, note type, course, onset and offset dates, and whether present during past month (e.g., "bizarre delusions of being controlled by aliens, present intermittently, onset 1969, offset June 1993").

Type of symptom	Course	Onset	Offset	Check if present during past month
Persecutory delusions	several weeks	1/96		✓

C. DIFFERENTIAL DIAGNOSIS OF PSYCHOTIC DISORDERS

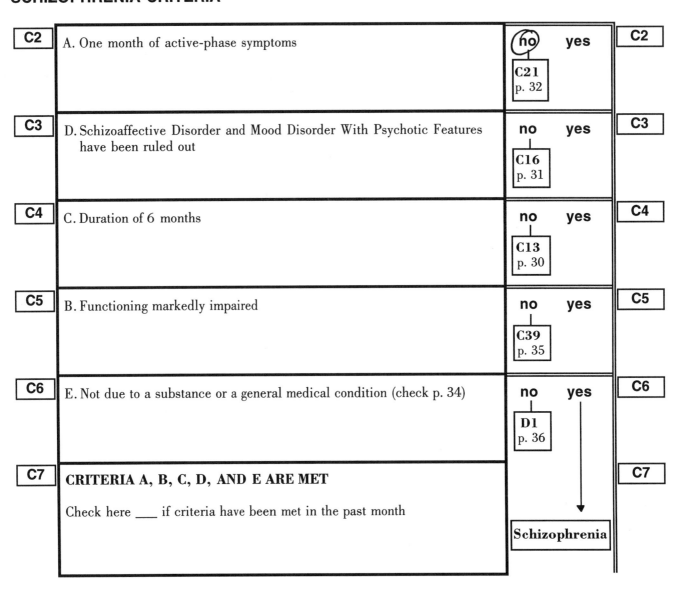

D1 p. 36			

C1 | Psychotic symptoms occur at times other than during mood episodes

no mood episodes | **no** (**yes**) | **C1**
D1 p. 36 | under "no"

SCHIZOPHRENIA CRITERIA

C2 | A. One month of active-phase symptoms | (**no**) **yes** — **C21** p. 32 | **C2**

C3 | D. Schizoaffective Disorder and Mood Disorder With Psychotic Features have been ruled out | **no** **yes** — **C16** p. 31 | **C3**

C4 | C. Duration of 6 months | **no** **yes** — **C13** p. 30 | **C4**

C5 | B. Functioning markedly impaired | **no** **yes** — **C39** p. 35 | **C5**

C6 | E. Not due to a substance or a general medical condition (check p. 34) | **no** **yes** — **D1** p. 36 | **C6**

C7 | **CRITERIA A, B, C, D, AND E ARE MET**

Check here ____ if criteria have been met in the past month | → **Schizophrenia** | **C7**

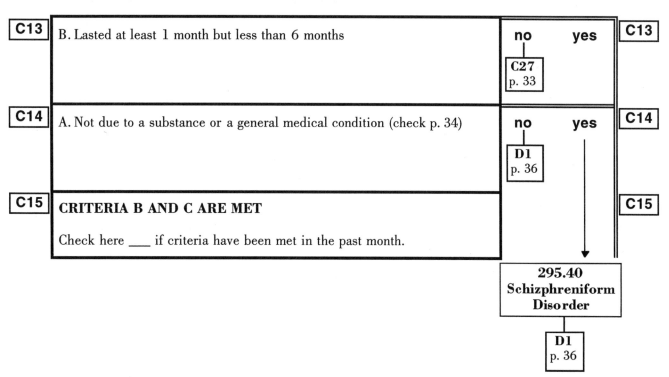

		no	yes	
C8	295.30 Schizophrenia, Paranoid Type		D1 p. 36	**C8**
C9	295.20 Schizophrenia, Catatonic Type		D1 p. 36	**C9**
C10	295.10 Schizophrenia, Disorganized Type		D1 p. 36	**C10**
C11	295.90 Schizophrenia, Undifferentiated Type		D1 p. 36	**C11**
C12	295.60 Schizophrenia, Residual Type		D1 p. 36	**C12**

SCHIZOPHRENIFORM DISORDER CRITERIA

		no	yes	
C13	B. Lasted at least 1 month but less than 6 months	C27 p. 33		**C13**
C14	A. Not due to a substance or a general medical condition (check p. 34)	D1 p. 36	↓	**C14**
C15	**CRITERIA B AND C ARE MET** Check here ___ if criteria have been met in the past month.			**C15**

295.40 Schizphreniform Disorder

D1 p. 36

SCHIZOAFFECTIVE DISORDER CRITERIA

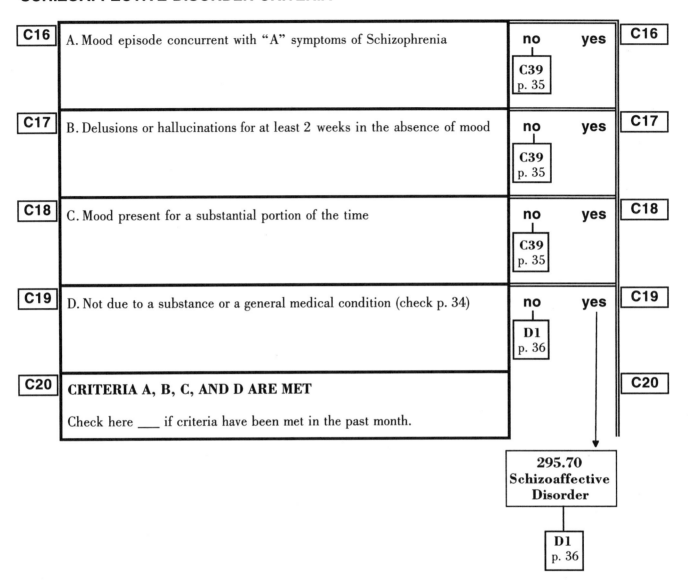

C16	A. Mood episode concurrent with "A" symptoms of Schizophrenia	**no** **yes** C39 p. 35	**C16**
C17	B. Delusions or hallucinations for at least 2 weeks in the absence of mood	**no** **yes** C39 p. 35	**C17**
C18	C. Mood present for a substantial portion of the time	**no** **yes** C39 p. 35	**C18**
C19	D. Not due to a substance or a general medical condition (check p. 34)	**no** **yes** D1 p. 36	**C19**
C20	**CRITERIA A, B, C, AND D ARE MET** Check here ___ if criteria have been met in the past month.		**C20**

295.70 Schizoaffective Disorder

D1 p. 36

DELUSIONAL DISORDER CRITERIA

C21	A. Nonbizarre delusions FBI guy	no · (yes) C27 p. 33	C21
C22	B. Never met criterion A for Schizophrenia	no · (yes) C39 p. 35	C22
C23	C. Functioning not odd or bizarre	no · (yes) C39 p. 35	C23
C24	D. Mood episodes brief relative to delusions	no · (yes) C39 p. 35	C24
C25	E. Not due to a substance or a general medical condition (check p. 34)	no · (yes) D1 p. 36	C25
C26	**CRITERIA A, B, C, D, AND E ARE MET** Check here ✓ if criteria have been met in the past month.		C26

297.1
Delusional
Disorder

D1
p. 36

Role-Play—Case 4

"Junior Executive"

OVERVIEW: [Read this to the interviewer] A 28-year-old female junior executive is referred for psychotherapy by her family physician. She complained to him of being "depressed about everything"—her job, her husband, and her prospects for the future.

MOOD SYMPTOMS: In response to the initial question about depressed mood, say you have been depressed almost as long as you can remember—at least since high school. To loss of interest or pleasure, say you get very little pleasure out of anything you do. Insist that this is nearly every day. When asked about appetite (criterion A2), say that when you are feeling really bad, you eat all day. If the interviewer asks if it is nearly every day, say "no, maybe 2 or 3 days a week in the past month." Say "no" to sleep problems or sleeping too much (criterion A4) and to psychomotor agitation or retardation (criterion A5). In response to the energy question (criterion A6), say you feel tired all the time. To how you feel about yourself (criterion A7), say you are disappointed about not being promoted, even though you do not really like your job but deny feelings of worthlessness or guilt. Say "no" to poor concentration (criterion A8) and suicide thoughts (criterion A9).

The interviewer should ask if you have had another time when you were depressed and had even more of these symptoms. Patiently explain that you have already said that is the way you always are.

Answer "no" to all the manic questions.

The interviewer will then ask you about the past 2 years. If he or she has been listening, this will hopefully be just a confirming question, such as "It sounds like you've been bothered by depressed mood more days than not in the past 2 years," to which you answer "yes."

Answer "yes" to overeating, low energy, low self-esteem, and feelings of hopelessness.

In response to what is the longest time you have felt okay, say never more than a week or two.

Deny medical illness or substance use.

PSYCHOTIC AND ASSOCIATED SYMPTOMS: Say "no" to everything.

> *SCID Diagnosis:*
>   Dysthymic Disorder
> *GAF:* 58
>   (moderate symptoms—depressed mood, fatigue, anhedonia, overeating)

Role-Play—Case 5

"Drug Store"

OVERVIEW: [Read this to the interviewer] This 40-year-old swimming pool contractor who lives alone is interviewed in a community study. He has never been in treatment. He is currently in the midst of his busy season, working 60 hours a week, and spending evenings at the hospital visiting his terminally ill mother.

MOOD SYMPTOMS: Answer "yes" to the depression question, but when the interviewer asks about "most of the day, nearly every day," say "no;" you are depressed about your mother, but you do not think about it during the day because you are so busy. In response to loss of interest, say you do not have time to do anything but work, visit your mother, and sleep. If the interviewer (incorrectly) asks the Major Depressive Episode questions, answer "no" to all of them. Answer "no" to the manic and dysthymic questions in the mood module.

PSYCHOTIC AND ASSOCIATED SYMPTOMS: Answer "no" to everything, except for vivid brightly colored "auras" (visual illusions—*not* hallucinations) when you were high on LSD.

SUBSTANCE USE DISORDERS: In response to the questions regarding your drinking habits, say that you usually drink two glasses of wine with dinner, or three or four beers during a social evening. If the interviewer decides to ask you about alcohol abuse, you should answer "no" to all the questions.

About drugs, here is your history of pattern of use in response to the question on page 58 of the Administration Booklet referring you to the "drug list." Between ages 25 and 35 you used drugs in the following pattern:

1. You smoked **marijuana** occasionally, usually on weekends, for most of this 10-year period. There was no period of particularly heavy use.
2. When it was available, sometimes for months at a time (because you were dealing it), you snorted **cocaine** daily. You remember that the period of heaviest use was around age 31 for about 6 months.
3. You used **Quaaludes** when you were with a girlfriend who had a supplier because they were great for sex (heaviest use—twice a week for 4 months age 27).
4. Sporadically, you have also used **amphetamines** (when you had to drive long distances and needed to stay awake).
5. You have used **hallucinogens** (LSD) maybe 20 times over the 10 years and have used mescaline and "mushrooms" occasionally.

The interviewer should ask you all of the Substance Dependence questions for cocaine, because that drug was the most heavily used and most likely to have caused Dependence. Answer "yes" to the first question (criterion 3—use of larger amount than intended), saying that you often used up all your cocaine in one evening, even when you had an amount that should last for a week. Also answer "yes" to the second question (criterion 4—persistent desire or several attempts to quit)—you tried to stop many times but succeeded only when you moved to a place where it was not easy to get. To question #3 (criterion 5—a lot of time spent), ask the interviewer what he or she means by "a lot of time," then say you were often "coked up" at work. For criterion 6 (activities given up), answer "no." For criterion 7 (continued use despite knowledge of problem), explain that the coke made you paranoid at work, and you kept using it anyway. For criterion 1 (tolerance), you needed to escalate the amount of cocaine you used. Finally, (criterion 2) report that when you finally quit cocaine you were irritable, were exhausted, and had trouble sleeping for weeks.

SCID Diagnosis:
   Cocaine Dependence, Lifetime (not current)
GAF: 75
   (depression in response to mother's illness)

S C I D - I

CLINICIAN VERSION

SCORESHEET

Michael B. First, M.D.
Robert L. Spitzer, M.D.
Miriam Gibbon, M.S.W.
Janet B. W. Williams, D.S.W.

Biometrics Research Department
New York State Psychiatric Institute
Department of Psychiatry
Columbia University
New York, New York

Patient's name: _____Drug   Store_____

Record number: ___301_____   Date of evaluation: __6/2/94___

Clinician: __First___

Sources of information (check all that apply):   ☒ Patient
   ❑ Family/friends/associates
   ❑ Health professional
   ❑ Medical records

SUBSTANCE USE DISORDERS

Current	Lifetime		**Alcohol Use Disorders**
❏	❏	303.90	Alcohol Dependence (*E15*, p. 42)
❏	❏	305.00	Alcohol Abuse (*E16*, p. 42)

Other Substance Use Disorders

Current	Lifetime		
❏	❏	304.90	Amphetamine Dependence (*E31*, p. 46)
❏	❏	304.30	Cannabis Dependence (*E31*, p. 46)
❏	☒	304.20	Cocaine Dependence (*E31*, p. 46)
❏	❏	304.50	Hallucinogen Dependence (*E31*, p. 46)
❏	❏	304.60	Inhalant Dependence (*E31*, p. 46)
❏	❏	304.00	Opioid Dependence (*E31*, p. 46)
❏	❏	304.60	Phencyclidine Dependence (*E31*, p. 46)
❏	❏	304.10	Sedative, Hypnotic, or Anxiolytic Dependence (*E31*, p. 46)
❏	❏	304.90	Other (or Unknown) Substance Dependence (*E31*, p. 46)
❏	❏	305.70	Amphetamine Abuse (*E32*, p. 46)
❏	❏	305.20	Cannabis Abuse (*E32*, p. 46)
❏	❏	305.60	Cocaine Abuse (*E32*, p. 46)
❏	❏	305.30	Hallucinogen Abuse (*E32*, p. 46)
❏	❏	305.90	Inhalant Abuse (*E32*, p. 46)
❏	❏	305.50	Opioid Abuse (*E32*, p. 46)
❏	❏	305.90	Phencyclidine Abuse (*E32*, p. 46)
❏	❏	305.40	Sedative, Hypnotic, or Anxiolytic Abuse (*E32*, p. 46)
❏	❏	305.90	Other (or Unknown) Substance Use (*E32*, p. 46)

ANXIETY DISORDERS

Current	Lifetime		
❏	❏	300.21	Panic Disorder With Agoraphobia (*F23*, p. 49)
❏	❏	300.01	Panic Disorder Without Agoraphobia (*F24*, p. 49)
❏	❏	300.3	Obsessive-Compulsive Disorder (*F38*, p. 52)
❏	❏	309.81	Posttraumatic Stress Disorder (*F64*, p. 56)
❏	❏	300.0	Anxiety Disorder Not Otherwise Specified (*F71*, p. 57)
❏	❏	293.84	Anxiety Disorder Due to a General Medical Condition (*F86*, p. 60)

Indicate General Medical Condition: _____

check specifier:

___ With Generalized Anxiety

___ With Panic Attacks

___ With Obsessive-Compulsive Symptoms

E. ALCOHOL AND OTHER SUBSTANCE USE DISORDERS

E7
p. 41

| E1 | Had a period of excessive drinking OR had evidence of alcohol-related problems | ?   —   ⊕ | E1 |

E17
p. 43

ALCOHOL ABUSE CRITERIA

A. A maladaptive pattern of alcohol use leading to clinically significant impairment or distress, as manifested by one (or more) of the following occurring within a 12-month period:

E2	(1) failure to fulfill major role obligations at work, school, or home *Notes:*	? ⊖ +	E2
E3	(2) use in situations in which it is physically hazardous *Notes:*	? ⊖ +	E3
E4	(3) recurrent alcohol-related legal problems *Notes:*	? ⊖ +	E4
E5	(4) continued alcohol use despite having problems caused or exacerbated by the effects of alcohol *Notes:*	? ⊖ +	E5
E6	**AT LEAST ONE ABUSE ITEM IS "+"**	? ⊖ +	E6

E17
p. 43

Ratings: ? = Inadequate information;   − = Absent (or subthreshold);   + = Present

NONALCOHOL SUBSTANCE USE DISORDERS

| E17 | CIRCLE THE NAME OF EACH DRUG EVER USED (OR WRITE IN NAME IF "OTHER"). | RECORD PERIOD OF HEAVIEST USE (AGE OR DATE, AND DURATION) AND DESCRIBE PATTERN OF USE. | E17 |

CIRCLE THE NAME OF EACH DRUG EVER USED (OR WRITE IN NAME IF "OTHER").	RECORD PERIOD OF HEAVIEST USE (AGE OR DATE, AND DURATION) AND DESCRIBE PATTERN OF USE.
Sedatives-hypnotics-anxiolytics: (Quaalude,) Seconal, Valium, Xanax, Librium, barbiturates, Miltown, Ativan, Dalmane, Halcion, Restoril, or other: _____	Age 27 — twice a week, 4 months
Cannabis: (marijuana,) hashish, THC, or other: _____	Ages 25–35 — occasionally on weekends
Stimulants: (amphetamine,) "speed," crystal meth, dexadrine, Ritalin, "ice," or other: _____	Occasionally to stay awake on long drives
Opioids: heroin, morphine, opium, Methadone, Darvon, codeine, Percodan, Demerol, Dilaudid, unspecified or other: _____	
Cocaine: (intranasal,) IV, freebase, crack, "speedball," unspecified or other: _____	Age 31 — daily for at least 6 months — dealing it
Hallucinogens/PCP: (LSD,) (mescaline,) peyote, psilocybin, STP, (mushrooms,) PCP ("angel dust"), Special K (ketamine), Extasy, MDMA, or other: _____	LSD 20 times over 10 years Mescaline + mushrooms occasionally
Other: steroids, "glue," paint, inhalants, nitrous oxide ("laughing gas"), amyl or butyl nitrate ("poppers"), nonprescription sleep or diet pills, unknown, or other: _____	

DRUG CLASS USED MOST/MOST PROBLEMS:

Cocaine _____

| E23 p. 45 | | if "NONE" F1, p. 47 |

NONALCOHOL SUBSTANCE DEPENDENCE CRITERIA

A maladaptive pattern of substance use, leading to clinically significant impairment or distress, as manifested by three (or more) of the following occurring at any time in the same 12-month period:

Cocaine

E23 (3) often taken in larger amounts OR over a longer period than was intended
Notes: used up 1 week's supply in one evening
? — ⊕ **E23**

E24 (4) there is a persistent desire OR unsuccessful effort to cut down or control substance
Notes: tried to stop many times — able to only when couldn't get it any more
? — ⊕ **E24**

E25 (5) a great deal of time is spent in activities necessary to obtain substance, use it, or recover from its effects
Notes: high at work and on weekends
? — ⊕ **E25**

E26 (6) important social, occupational, or recreational activities given up or reduced because of use
Notes:
? ⊖ + **E26**

E27 (7) continued use despite knowledge of having a persistent or recurrent physical or psychological problem
Notes: made him "paranoid"
? — ⊕ **E27**

Ratings: ? = Inadequate information;   — = Absent (or subthreshold);   + = Present

E28	(1) tolerance *Notes:* Steady escalation in amount needed	? — ⊕	E28
E29	(2) withdrawal *Notes:* irritable, fatigue, insomnia	? — ⊕	E29
E30	**AT LEAST THREE DEPENDENCE ITEMS ARE "+" AND OCCURRED WITHIN THE SAME 12-MONTH PERIOD**	? — ⊕ E18, p. 44 E32, below	E30

| E31 | Check:
___ **304.90 Amphetamine Dependence**
___ **304.30 Cannabis Dependence**
X **304.20 Cocaine Dependence**
___ **304.50 Hallucinogen Dependence**
___ **304.60 Inhalant Dependence**
___ **304.00 Opioid Dependence**
___ **304.60 Phencyclidine Dependence**
___ **304.10 Sedative, Hypnotic, or Anxiolytic Dependence**
___ **304.90 Other (or Unknown) Substance Dependence**
Check here ___ if criteria have been met in the past month. | ⊕
↓
Substance Dependence
F1
p. 47 | E31 |
| E32 | Check:
___ **305.70 Amphetamine Abuse**
___ **305.20 Cannabis Abuse**
___ **305.60 Cocaine Abuse**
___ **305.30 Hallucinogen Abuse**
___ **305.90 Inhalant Abuse**
___ **305.50 Opioid Abuse**
___ **305.90 Phencyclidine Abuse**
___ **305.40 Sedative, Hypnotic, or Anxiolytic Abuse**
___ **305.90 Other (or Unknown) Substance Use**
Check here ___ if criteria have been met in the past month. | +
↓
Substance Abuse
F1
p. 47 | E32 |

Ratings: **? = Inadequate information;**   **– = Absent (or subthreshold);**   **+ = Present**

Role-Play—Case 6

"Panic at the Airport"

OVERVIEW: [Read this to the interviewer] This 37-year-old married mother of two small children is referred for an evaluation after a negative medical workup. One year ago she had what she thought was a heart attack while waiting at the airport for her parents to arrive. Since then, she has had many such attacks and is now unwilling to leave the house except for medical appointments.

MOOD SYMPTOMS: Answer "no" to all screening questions.

PSYCHOTIC AND ASSOCIATED SYMPTOMS: Answer "no" to all questions.

SUBSTANCE USE DISORDERS: You drink rarely, only a ceremonial glass of champagne at weddings and so forth. You have never used illegal drugs nor had any problem with prescribed drugs.

ANXIETY AND OTHER DISORDERS: When asked about panic attacks, say that doctors tell you that is what they are. You have had many of them, sometimes three or four times a day. When asked if they come unexpectedly, say "yes." The interviewer will then ask whether you worry that there is something wrong with you. Say that at first you worried that it was a heart attack. Now you guess you believe them that it is not your heart, but the experience is so overwhelming that you are afraid to go anywhere because you never can tell when you'll have one.

When asked to describe the last bad one, say it was just this morning. You were getting dressed when all of a sudden you felt nauseous and dizzy and like something terrible was going to happen. Then you got very hot and began to sweat. It lasted about 15 minutes.

When the interviewer reads the symptom list, answer "yes" to palpitations, sweating, trembling, nausea, dizziness, fear of losing control, and hot flashes and "no" to other symptoms. In response to questions about being physically ill or using drugs, say "no."

In response to the question about situations that make you nervous, say you do not feel safe unless you are at home or in a doctor's office. You could have an attack anywhere, and you need either your husband or a doctor with you to take care of you.

Answer "no" to the question about thoughts that do not make sense but "yes" to the one about doing things over and over. Explain that you have always had this ridiculous ritual: when you take a garment out of a drawer you have to shake it 10 times to make sure there are no mice nesting in it. (You once did find a nest of baby mice in your drawer and it freaked you out.) When asked whether you do it more than makes sense, answer that of course it does not make sense. It is ridiculous. In response to what effect it has on your life, say "very little" . . . it's just annoying, and it only takes you a few extra minutes, but you feel uncomfortable if you do not do it.

SCID Diagnosis:
   Panic Disorder, With Agoraphobia
GAF: 36
   (the panic attacks and Agoraphobia cause major impairment in functioning)

STRUCTURED CLINICAL INTERVIEW FOR DSM-IV AXIS I DISORDERS

S C I D - I

CLINICIAN VERSION

SCORESHEET

Michael B. First, M.D.
Robert L. Spitzer, M.D.
Miriam Gibbon, M.S.W.
Janet B. W. Williams, D.S.W.

Biometrics Research Department
New York State Psychiatric Institute
Department of Psychiatry
Columbia University
New York, New York

Patient's name: __Panic at the Airport__

Record number: __333__   Date of evaluation: __2/8/92__

Clinician: __Gibbon__

Sources of information (check all that apply): ☒ Patient

☐ Family/friends/associates

☐ Health professional

☐ Medical records

SUBSTANCE USE DISORDERS

Current	Lifetime			
		Alcohol Use Disorders		
☐	☐	303.90	Alcohol Dependence (*E15*, p. 42)	
☐	☐	305.00	Alcohol Abuse (*E16*, p. 42)	
		Other Substance Use Disorders		
☐	☐	304.90	Amphetamine Dependence (*E31*, p. 46)	
☐	☐	304.30	Cannabis Dependence (*E31*, p. 46)	
☐	☐	304.20	Cocaine Dependence (*E31*, p. 46)	
☐	☐	304.50	Hallucinogen Dependence (*E31*, p. 46)	
☐	☐	304.60	Inhalant Dependence (*E31*, p. 46)	
☐	☐	304.00	Opioid Dependence (*E31*, p. 46)	
☐	☐	304.60	Phencyclidine Dependence (*E31*, p. 46)	
☐	☐	304.10	Sedative, Hypnotic, or Anxiolytic Dependence (*E31*, p. 46)	
☐	☐	304.90	Other (or Unknown) Substance Dependence (*E31*, p. 46)	
☐	☐	305.70	Amphetamine Abuse (*E32*, p. 46)	
☐	☐	305.20	Cannabis Abuse (*E32*, p. 46)	
☐	☐	305.60	Cocaine Abuse (*E32*, p. 46)	
☐	☐	305.30	Hallucinogen Abuse (*E32*, p. 46)	
☐	☐	305.90	Inhalant Abuse (*E32*, p. 46)	
☐	☐	305.50	Opioid Abuse (*E32*, p. 46)	
☐	☐	305.90	Phencyclidine Abuse (*E32*, p. 46)	
☐	☐	305.40	Sedative, Hypnotic, or Anxiolytic Abuse (*E32*, p. 46)	
☐	☐	305.90	Other (or Unknown) Substance Use (*E32*, p. 46)	

ANXIETY DISORDERS

Current	Lifetime		
☒	☒	300.21	Panic Disorder With Agoraphobia (*F23*, p. 49)
☐	☐	300.01	Panic Disorder Without Agoraphobia (*F24*, p. 49)
☐	☐	300.3	Obsessive-Compulsive Disorder (*F38*, p. 52)
☐	☐	309.81	Posttraumatic Stress Disorder (*F64*, p. 56)
☐	☐	300.0	Anxiety Disorder Not Otherwise Specified (*F71*, p. 57)
☐	☐	293.84	Anxiety Disorder Due to a General Medical Condition (*F86*, p. 60)

Indicate General Medical Condition: _____

check specifier:

___ With Generalized Anxiety
___ With Panic Attacks
___ With Obsessive-Compulsive Symptoms

F. ANXIETY AND OTHER DISORDERS

PANIC DISORDER CRITERIA

F1	A. (1) recurrent unexpected panic attacks *Notes:* first one a year ago—now has them 3-4 times a day Completely unpredictable—at home & outside	? — ⊕ F25 p. 50	**F1**
F2	A. (2) at least one of the following: (b) worry about the implications of the attack; (a) concern about having additional attacks; (c) a <u>significant</u> <u>change in behavior</u> *Notes:* housebound	? — ⊕ F25 p. 50	**F2**
F3	Four (or more) of the following panic attack symptoms developed abruptly and reached a peak within 10 minutes *Notes:*	? — ⊕ F25 p. 50	**F3**
F4	(1) palpitations	? — ⊕	**F4**
F5	(2) sweating	? — ⊕	**F5**
F6	(3) trembling or shaking	? — ⊕	**F6**
F7	(4) shortness of breath	? ⊖ +	**F7**
F8	(5) choking	? ⊖ +	**F8**
F9	(6) chest pain	? ⊖ +	**F9**
F10	(7) nausea or abdominal distress	? — ⊕	**F10**
F11	(8) feeling dizzy	? — ⊕	**F11**
F12	(9) derealization or depersonalization	? ⊖ +	**F12**
F13	(10) fear of losing control or going crazy	? — ⊕	**F13**
F14	(11) fear of dying	? ⊖ +	**F14**
F15	(12) paresthesias	? ⊖ +	**F15**
F16	(13) chills or hot flashes	? — ⊕	**F16**

Ratings: ? = Inadequate information;   – = Absent (or subthreshold);   + = Present

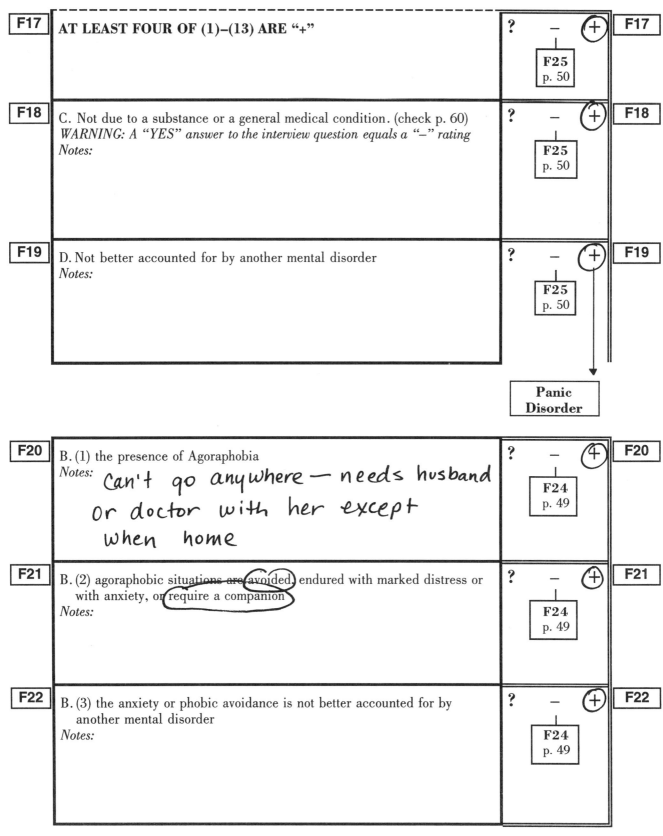

| F17 | AT LEAST FOUR OF (1)–(13) ARE "+" | ? — ⊕   F25 p. 50 | F17 |

| F18 | C. Not due to a substance or a general medical condition. (check p. 60) *WARNING: A "YES" answer to the interview question equals a "–" rating* Notes: | ? — ⊕   F25 p. 50 | F18 |

| F19 | D. Not better accounted for by another mental disorder Notes: | ? — ⊕   F25 p. 50 | F19 |

Panic Disorder

| F20 | B. (1) the presence of Agoraphobia Notes: *Can't go anywhere — needs husband or doctor with her except when home* | ? — ④   F24 p. 49 | F20 |

| F21 | B. (2) agoraphobic situations are avoided, endured with marked distress or with anxiety, or require a companion Notes: | ? — ⊕   F24 p. 49 | F21 |

| F22 | B. (3) the anxiety or phobic avoidance is not better accounted for by another mental disorder Notes: | ? — ⊕   F24 p. 49 | F22 |

Ratings: **? = Inadequate information;**   **– = Absent (or subthreshold);**   **+ = Present**

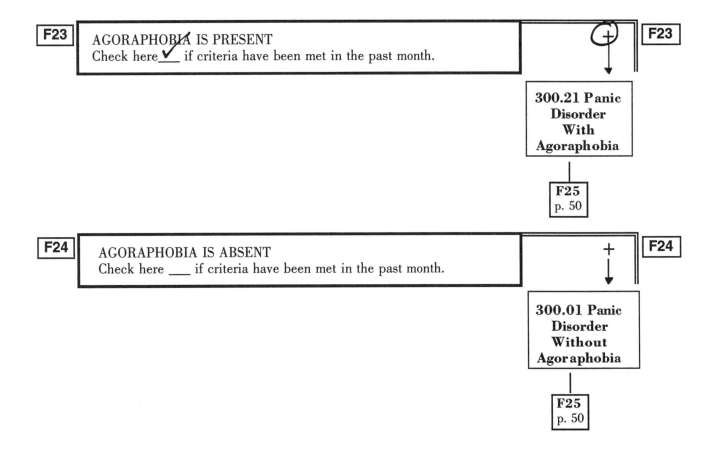

| F23 | AGORAPHOBIA IS PRESENT
Check here ✔ if criteria have been met in the past month. | ⊕ | F23 |

300.21 Panic Disorder With Agoraphobia

F25 p. 50

| F24 | AGORAPHOBIA IS ABSENT
Check here ___ if criteria have been met in the past month. | + | F24 |

300.01 Panic Disorder Without Agoraphobia

F25 p. 50

Ratings: ? = Inadequate information;   − = Absent (or subthreshold);   + = Present

OBSESSIVE-COMPULSIVE DISORDER CRITERIA

F25	*Obsessions:* (1) recurrent and persistent thoughts, impulses, or images *Notes:*	? ⊖ + F30 below	F25
F26	(2) not simply excessive worries about real-life problems *Notes:*	? − + F30 below	F26
F27	(3) the person attempts to ignore or suppress or neutralize such thoughts *Notes:*	? − + F30 below	F27
F28	(4) the person recognizes that they are a product of his or her own mind *Notes:*	? − + F30 below	F28
F29	**OBSESSIONS (1), (2), (3), AND (4) ARE "+"**	? − +	F29
F30	*Compulsions:* (1) repetitive behaviors or mental acts *Notes:* need to shake garments 10 times when she takes them out of drawer	? − ⊕ F33 p. 51	F30

Ratings: ? = Inadequate information;   − = Absent (or subthreshold);   + = Present

F31	(2) the behaviors or mental acts are aimed at preventing or reducing distress *Notes:* to make sure no mouse nest!	? − ⊕ F33 below	F31
F32	**COMPULSIONS (1) AND (2) ARE "+"**	? − ⊕	F32
F33	**EITHER F29 IS "+" OR F32 IS "+"** (i.e., either obsessions or compulsions)	? − ⊕ F39 p. 52	F33
F34	B. The person has recognized that the obsessions or compulsions are excessive or unreasonable. *Notes:* Doesn't make any sense	? − ⊕ F39 p. 52	F34
F35	C. The obsessions or compulsions are clinically significant. *Notes:* Very little time spent	? ⊖ + F39 p. 52	F35
F36	D. If another Axis I disorder is present, the content of the obsessions or compulsions is not restricted to it. *Notes:*	? − + F39 p. 52	F36

Ratings: **? = Inadequate information;**   **− = Absent (or subthreshold);**   **+ = Present**

Homework—Case 1

"Low Life Level"

Louise Larkin is a pale, stooped woman age 39 years, whose childlike face is surrounded by scraggly blond braids tied with pink ribbons. She was referred for a psychiatric evaluation for possible hospitalization by her family physician who was concerned about her low level of functioning. Her only complaint to him was: "I have a decline in self-care and a low life level." Her mother reports that there has indeed been a decline but that it has been over many years. In the past few months, she has remained in her room, mute and still.

Twelve years ago, Louise was a supervisor in the occupational therapy department of a large hospital, living in her own apartment, and was engaged to a young man. He broke the engagement, and she became increasingly disorganized, wandering aimlessly in the street, wearing mismatched clothing. She was fired from her job, and eventually the police were called to hospitalize her. They broke into her apartment, which was in shambles and filled with papers, food, and broken objects. No information is available from this hospitalization, which lasted 3 months and from which she was discharged to her mother's house with a prescription for unknown medication that she never had filled.

After her discharge, her family hoped that she would gather herself together and embark again on a real life, but as the years progressed she became more withdrawn and less functional. Most of her time was spent watching television and cooking. Her cooking consisted of mixing bizarre combinations of ingredients, such as broccoli and cake mix, and cooking and eating them alone because no one else in the family would eat her meals. She collected cookbooks and recipes, cluttering her room with stacks of these. Often when her mother entered her room, she would quickly grab a magazine and pretend to be reading, when in fact she had apparently just been sitting and staring into space. She stopped bathing and brushing her hair or teeth. She ate less and less, although she denied loss of appetite, and over a period of several years lost 20 pounds. She would sleep at odd hours. Eventually she became enuretic, wetting her bed frequently and filling the room with the pungent odor of urine.

On admission to the psychiatric hospital she sat with her hands tightly clasped in her lap and avoided looking at the physician who interviewed her. She answered questions readily and did not appear suspicious or guarded, but her affect was shallow. She denied depressed mood, delusions, or hallucinations. However, her answers became increasingly idiosyncratic and irrelevant as the interview progressed. In response to a question about her strange cooking habits, she replied that she did not wish to discuss recent events in Russia. When discussing her decline in functioning, she said, "There's more of a take-off mechanism when you're younger." Asked about ideas of reference, she said, "I doubt it's true, but if one knows the writers involved, it could be an element that would be directed in a comical way." Her answers were interspersed with the mantra, "I'm safe. I'm safe."

SCID Coding for "Low Life Level"

Module A:

Page 13:   A1 = "–"; A2 = "–"

Page 15:   A16 = "–"

Page 21:   A45 = "–"

Module B:

Page 26:   B1 through B7 = "–"

Page 27:   B8 through B10 = "–"
          B11 = "+" (*Grossly disorganized be-havior*—"she became increas-ingly disorganized, wandering aimlessly in the street, wearing mismatched clothing")
          B12 = "–"
          B13 = "+" (*Disorganized speech*—"answers became increasingly idiosyncratic and irrele-vant" . . . "I doubt it's true, but if one knows the writers involved, it could be an ele-ment that would be directed in a comical way")
          B14 = "+" (Negative symptoms: *Avolition*—"sitting and staring into space" . . . "stopped brushing her hair or teeth")

Module C:

Page 29:   C1   = "yes" (psychotic symptoms outside of Mood Episodes)
           C2   = "yes" (disorganized speech and negative symptoms occur-ring together for at least a month)
           C3   = "yes" (no mood episode ever)
           C4   = "yes" (continuous signs of ill-ness for years)
           C5   = "yes" (severe functional im-pairment)
           C6   = "yes" (not due to general medical condition or sub-stance)
           C7   = (criteria A, B, C, D, and E are met) Criteria met in the past month
           C8   = "no" (no delusions or halluci-nations)

Page 30:   C9   = "no" (no catatonic symptoms)
           C10 = "no" (disorganized behavior not present along with dis-organized speech)
           C11 = "yes" (Undifferentiated Type)

SCID Diagnosis:
295.90 Schizophrenia, Undifferentiated Type,
    Current
GAF: 15
    (occasionally fails to maintain personal hygiene)

Homework—Case 2

"I Am Vishnu"

Mr. Nehru is a 32-year-old, single, unemployed man who migrated from India to the United States when he was 13. His brother brought him to the emergency department of an Atlanta, Georgia, hospital after neighbors complained that he was standing in the street harassing people about his religious beliefs. To the psychiatrist he keeps repeating, "I am Vishnu. I am Krishna."

Mr. Nehru has been living with his brother and sister-in-law for the past 7 months, attending an outpatient clinic. During the past 4 weeks, his behavior has become increasingly disruptive. He awakens his brother at all hours of the night to discuss religious matters. He often seems to be responding to voices that only he hears. He neither bathes nor changes his clothes.

Mr. Nehru's first episode of emotional disturbance was 5 years ago. Medical records are not available, but from the brother's account it seems to have been similar to the present episode. There have been two other similar episodes, each requiring hospitalization for a few months. Mr. Nehru admits that, starting about 5 years previously and virtually continuously since then, he has been troubled by "voices" that he hears throughout the day. There are several voices, which comment on his behavior and discuss him in the third person. They usually are either benign ("Look at him now. He is about to eat.") or insulting in content ("What a fool he is. He doesn't understand anything!").

Between episodes, according to both his outpatient psychiatrist and his brother, Mr. Nehru is a quiet, somewhat withdrawn person who is popular in his neighborhood because he helps some of his elderly neighbors with shopping and yard work. At these times his mood is unremarkable. However, he claims that because of the "voices," he cannot concentrate sufficiently to hold a job. He sometimes reads books but watches little television because he hears the voices coming out of the television and is upset that the television shows often refer to him.

For the past 6 weeks, with increasing insistence, the voices have been telling Mr. Nehru that he is the new Messiah, Jesus, Moses, Vishnu, and Krishna and should begin a new religious epoch in human history. He has begun to experience surges of increased energy, "so I could spread my gospel," and needs very little sleep. According to his brother, he has become more preoccupied with the voices and disorganized in his daily activities.

When interviewed, Mr. Nehru is euphoric, and his speech is rapid and hard to follow. He paces up and down the ward and, on seeing a physician, grabs his arm, puts his face within 2 inches of the physician's, and talks with great rapidity and enthusiasm about his religious "insights." In the middle of a speech on his new religion, he abruptly compliments the physician on how well his shirt and tie match. When limits are placed on his behavior, he becomes loud and angry. In addition to his belief that he is the Messiah, he feels that the hospital is part of a conspiracy to suppress his religious message. Although he seems to enjoy his "voices," he sometimes complains about them and makes references to "those damned voices." He states that he feels that his religious insights, euphoria, and energy have been put into him by God.

SCID Coding for "I Am Vishnu"

Module A:

Page 13: A1 =   "–"; A2 = "–"

Page 15: A16 =   "+" ("Mr. Nehru is euphoric")

              A17 =   "+" (hospitalized)

              A18 =   "+" ("he is the new Messiah")

Page 16: A19 =   "+" ("needs very little sleep")

              A20 =   "+" ("talks with great rapidity and enthusiasm")

              A21 =   "+" ("speech is rapid and hard to follow")

              A22 =   "+" ("in the middle of a speech on his new religion, he abruptly compliments the physician on how well his shirt and tie match")

              A23 =   "+" ("he paces up and down the ward")

              A24 =   "–"

              A25 =   "+"

Page 17: A26 =   "+" (hospitalized)

              A27 =   "+" (not due to general medical condition or substance)

              A28 =   "+" (meets criteria for a Manic Episode) Criteria met in the past month

              A29 =   three Manic Episodes

Module B:

Page 26: B1 =   "+" ("the television shows often refer to him")

              B2 =   "+" ("the hospital is part of a conspiracy to suppress his religious message")

              B3 =   "+" ("he is the new Messiah")

              B4 and B5 = "–"

              B6 =   "+" ("troubled by voices that he hears throughout the day")

              B7 =   "–"

Page 27: B8 through B14 = "–"

Module C:

Page 29: C1 =   "yes" (psychotic symptoms when not manic—voices for 5 years)

              C2 =   "yes" (delusions and hallucinations)

              C3 =   "no" (there are manic symptoms concurrent with active phase symptoms of Schizophrenia, and total duration of the manic symptoms has not been brief relative to total duration of illness; manic symptoms accompany each exacerbation)

Page 31: C16 =   "yes" (manic symptoms concurrent with active phase symptoms of Schizophrenia)

              C17 =   "yes" (auditory hallucinations in the absence of prominent mood symptoms)

              C18 =   "yes" (Mood Episode symptoms for a substantial portion of the duration of the illness)

              C19 =   "yes" (not due to general medical condition/substance)

              C20 =   (criteria A, B, C, and D are met) Criteria met in the past month

---

SCID Diagnosis:
  295.70 Schizoaffective Disorder, Current
GAF: 17
  (occasionally fails to maintain personal hygiene—"neither bathes nor changes his clothes")

Homework—Case 3

"Contract on My Life"

Mr. Polsen, a 42-year-old married African American postal worker and father of two, is brought to the emergency department by his wife because he has been insisting that "there is a contract out on my life."

According to Mr. Polsen, his problems began 4 months ago when his supervisor at work accused him of tampering with a package. Mr. Polsen denied that this was true and, because his job was in jeopardy, filed a protest. At a formal hearing, he was exonerated and, according to him, "This made my boss furious. He felt he had been publicly humiliated."

About 2 weeks later, Mr. Polsen noticed that his co-workers were avoiding him. "When I'd walk toward them, they'd just turn away like they didn't want to see me." Shortly thereafter, he began to feel that they were talking about him at work. He never could make out clearly what they were saying, but he gradually became convinced that they were avoiding him because his boss had taken out a contract on his life.

This state of affairs was stable for about 2 months, until Mr. Polsen began noticing several "large white cars," new to his neighborhood, driving up and down the street on which he lived. He became increasingly frightened and was convinced that the "hit men" were in these cars. He refused to go out of his apartment without an escort. Several times, when he saw the white cars, he would panic and run home. After one such incident, his wife finally insisted that he accompany her to the emergency department.

Mr. Polsen was described by his wife and brother as a basically well-adjusted, outgoing man who enjoyed being with his family. He had served with distinction in Vietnam. He saw little combat there but was pulled from a burning truck by a buddy seconds before the truck blew up.

When interviewed, Mr. Polsen was obviously frightened. Aside from his belief that he was in danger of being killed, his speech, behavior, and demeanor were in no way odd or strange. His predominant mood was anxious. He denied having hallucinations and all other psychotic symptoms except those noted above. He claimed not to be depressed and, although he noted that he had recently had some difficulty falling asleep, he said there had been no change in his appetite, sex drive, energy level, or concentration.

SCID Coding for "Contract on My Life"

Module A:

Page 13: A1 =   "–"; A2 = "–"

Page 15: A16 = "–"

Page 21: A45 = "–"

Module B:

Page 26: B1 =   "+" ("hit men" in white cars;
                    co-workers turning away)
          B2 =   "+" (boss put out a contract on
                    his life)
          B3 through B7 = "–"
Page 27: B8 through B14 = "–"

Module C:

Page 29: C1 =   "yes" (no mood episodes)
          C2 =   "no" (no hallucinations, disor-
                    ganized speech or behavior or
                    negative symptoms)

Page 32: C21 = "yes" (nonbizarre delusion)
          C22 = "yes" (never met criteria for
                    Schizophrenia)
          C23 = "yes" (apart from impact of
                    delusion functioning not mark-
                    edly impaired; no odd or
                    bizarre behavior)
          C24 = "yes" (no Mood Episode ever)
          C25 = "yes" (not due to general
                    medical condition or
                    substance)
          C26 = (criteria A, B, C, D, and E are
                    met) Criteria have been pres-
                    ent in the past month

SCID Diagnosis:
  297.1 Delusional Disorder, Current
GAF: 27
  (behavior is markedly influenced by
  delusions—will not go out of apartment
  without an escort)

Homework—Case 4

"The Socialite"

Dorothea Cabot, a 42-year-old socialite, has never had any mental problems before. A new performance hall is to be formally opened with the world premiere of a new ballet, and Dorothea, because of her position on the cultural council, has assumed the responsibility for coordinating that event. However, construction problems, including strikes, have made it uncertain whether finishing details will meet the deadline. The set designer has been volatile, threatening to walk out on the project unless the materials meet his meticulous specifications. Dorothea has had to calm this volatile man while attempting to coax disputing groups to negotiate. She has also had increased responsibilities at home because her housekeeper has had to leave to visit a sick relative.

In the midst of these difficulties, her best friend was decapitated in a tragic auto crash. Dorothea herself is an only child, and her best friend had been close to her since grade school. People have often commented that the two women were like sisters.

Immediately following the funeral, Dorothea becomes increasingly tense and jittery and able to sleep only 2 to 3 hours a night. Two days later she happens to see a woman driving a car just like the one her friend had driven. She is puzzled, and after a few hours she becomes convinced that her friend is alive, that the accident had been staged, along with the funeral, as part of a plot. Somehow the plot is directed toward deceiving her, and she senses that somehow she is in great danger and must solve the mystery to escape alive. She begins to distrust everyone except her husband and begins to believe that the phone is tapped and that the rooms are "bugged." She pleads with her husband to help save her life. She begins to hear a high-pitched, undulating sound, which she fears is an ultrasound beam aimed at her. She is in a state of sheer panic, gripping her husband's arm in terror, as he brings her to the emergency department the next morning.

SCID Coding for "The Socialite"

Module A:

Page 13: A1 = "–"; A2 = "–"

Page 15: A16 = "–"

Page 21: A45 = "–"

Module B:

Page 26: B1 = "–"
            B2 = "+" (plot to deceive her; phone is tapped; room is bugged; she is in danger)
            B3 through B5 = "–"
            B6 = "+" (high-pitched "ultrasound")
            B7 = "–"

Page 27: B8 through B14 = "–"

Module C:

Page 29: C1 = "yes" (no Mood Episodes)
            C2 = "no" (both delusions and hallucinations but lasted less than 1 month)

Page 32: C21 = "no" (nonbizarre, but for less than 1 month)

Page 33: C27 = "yes" (delusions and hallucinations)
            C28 = "yes" (duration several days)
            C29 = "yes" (not better accounted for by another disorder)
            C30 = "yes" (not due to general medical condition or substance)
            C31 = (criteria A, B, and C are met) Criteria present in the past month

---

SCID Diagnosis:
   298.8 Brief Psychotic Disorder, Current
GAF: 25
   (behavior considerably influenced by delusions and hallucinations)

Homework—Case 5

"Under Surveillance"

Mr. Simpson is a 44-year-old, single, unemployed, white man brought into the emergency department by the police for striking an elderly woman in his apartment building. His chief complaint is, "That damn bitch. She and the rest of them deserved more than that for what they put me through."

He has been continuously ill since the age of 22. During his first year of law school, he gradually became more and more convinced that his classmates were making fun of him. He noticed that they would snort and sneeze whenever he entered the classroom. When a girl he was dating broke off the relationship with him, he believed that she had been "replaced" by a look-alike. He called the police and asked for their help to solve the "kidnapping." His academic performance in school declined dramatically, and he was asked to leave and seek psychiatric care.

Mr. Simpson got a job as an investment counselor at a bank, which he held for 7 months. However, he was getting an increasing number of distracting "signals" from co-workers, and he became more and more suspicious and withdrawn. It was at this time that he first reported hearing voices. He was eventually fired, and soon thereafter was hospitalized for the first time, at age 24. He has not worked since.

Mr. Simpson has been hospitalized 12 times, the longest stay being 8 months. However, in the past 5 years he has been hospitalized only once, for 3 weeks. During the hospitalizations he has received various antipsychotic drugs. Although outpatient medication has been prescribed, he usually stops taking it shortly after leaving the hospital. Aside from twice-yearly lunch meetings with his uncle and his contacts with mental health workers, he is totally isolated socially. He lives on his own and manages his own financial affairs, including a modest inheritance. He reads the *Wall Street Journal* daily. He cooks and cleans for himself.

Mr. Simpson maintains that his apartment is the center of a large communication system that involves all three major television networks, his neighbors, and apparently hundreds of "actors" in his neighborhood. There are secret cameras in his apartment that carefully monitor all his activities. When he is watching television, many of his minor actions (e.g., going to the bathroom) are soon directly commented on by the announcer. Whenever he goes outside, the "actors" have all been warned to keep him under surveillance. Everyone on the street watches him. His neighbors operate two different "machines"; one is responsible for all of his voices, except the "joker." He is not certain who controls this voice, which "visits" him only occasionally and is very funny. The other voices, which he hears many times each day, are generated by this machine, which he sometimes thinks is directly run by the neighbor whom he attacked. For example, when he is going over his investments, these "harassing" voices constantly tell him which stocks to buy. The other machine he calls "the dream machine." This machine puts erotic dreams into his head, usually of "black women."

Mr. Simpson describes other unusual experiences. For example, he recently went to a shoe store 30 miles from his house in the hope of getting some shoes that wouldn't be "altered." However, he soon found out that, like the rest of the shoes he buys, special nails had been put into the bottom of the shoes to annoy him. He was amazed that his decision concerning which shoe store to go to must have been known to his "harassers" before he himself knew it, so that they had time to get the altered shoes made up especially for him. He realizes that great effort and "millions of dollars" are involved in keeping him under surveillance. He sometimes thinks this is all part of a large experiment to discover the secret of his "superior intelligence."

At the interview, Mr. Simpson is well groomed, and his speech is coherent and goal-directed. His affect is, at most, only mildly blunted. He was initially angry at being brought in by the police. After several weeks of treatment with an antipsychotic drug failed to control his psychotic symptoms, he was transferred to a long-stay facility with the plan to arrange a structured living situation for him.

SCID coding for "Under Surveillance"

Module A:

Page 13: A1 =   "–"; A2 = "–"

Page 15: A16 = "–"

Page 21: A45 = "–"

Module B:

Page 26: B1 =   "+" (television comments on his behavior; everyone in the street watches him; shoes are "altered" to annoy him)

B2 =   "+" (machine-generated voices harass him)

B3 =   "+" (millions of dollars being spent, perhaps part of a large experiment to discover the secret of his superior intelligence)

B4 =   "–"

B5 =   "+" (girlfriend "replaced" by a look-alike; machine puts erotic dreams of black women in his head)

B6 =   "+" (machine-generated harassing voices every day)

B7 =   "–"

Page 27: B8 through B14 = "–"

Module C:

Page 29: C1 =   "yes" (no Mood Episode ever)

C2 =   "yes" (delusions and hallucinations for years)

C3 =   "yes" (no Mood Episode ever)

C4 =   "yes" (continuous signs of illness for years)

C5 =   "yes" (marked functional impairment)

C6 =   "yes" (not due to general medical condition or substance)

C7 =   (criteria A, B, C, D, and E are met) Criteria are met in the past month

C8 =   "yes" (preoccupied with delusions and hallucinations; no disorganized speech or behavior; no flat or inappropriate affect; no catatonic behavior)

SCID Diagnosis:
  295.30 Schizophrenia, Paranoid Type, Current
GAF: 20
  (behavior considerably influenced by psychotic symptoms, and some danger to others—hit elderly woman)

Homework—Case 6

"Agitated Businessman"

This agitated 42-year-old businessman was admitted to the psychiatric service after a $2^{1}/_{2}$-month period in which he found himself becoming increasingly distrustful of others and suspicious of his business associates. He was taking their statements out of context, "twisting" their words, and making inappropriately hostile and accusatory comments; he had, in fact, lost several business deals that had been "virtually sealed." Finally, the patient fired a shotgun into his backyard late one night when he heard noises that convinced him that intruders were about to break into his house and kill him.

One and one-half years previously, the patient had been diagnosed as having narcolepsy because of daily irresistible sleep attacks and episodes of sudden loss of muscle tone when he got emotionally excited and had been placed on an amphetamine-like stimulant, methylphenidate. He became asymptomatic and was able to work quite effectively as the sales manager of a small office-machine company and to participate in an active social life with his family and a small circle of friends.

In the 4 months before admission he had been using increasingly large doses of methylphenidate to maintain alertness late at night because of an increasing amount of work that could not be handled during the day. He reported that during this time he often could feel his heart race and had trouble sitting still.

SCID Coding for "Agitated Businessman"

Module A:

Page 13:   A1 =   "–"; A2 = "–"

Page 15:   A16 = "–"

Page 21:   A45 = "–"

Module B:

Page 26:   B1 =   "+" (he heard noises that convinced him that intruders were about to break into his house and kill him)

            B2 =   "–" (suspicious of business associates—not clear that he has a delusional conviction about any particular issue—remember to give the patient the benefit of the doubt when a psychotic symptom is not clearly present)

            B3 through B7 = "–"

Page 27:   B8 through B14 = "–"

Module C:

Page 29:   C1 =   "yes" (psychotic symptoms but no Mood Episodes)

            C2 =   "no" (only psychotic symptoms is a nonbizarre delusion of reference)

Page 32:   C21 = "yes" (nonbizarre delusion for 2 months)

            C22 = "yes" (has not met criterion A for Schizophrenia)

            C23 = "yes" (behavior not markedly impaired or bizarre)

            C24 = "yes" (no mood episodes)

The assessment of C25 requires that you first jump to page 34 (of the Scoresheet) to assess the etiology of the psychotic symptoms if there is a reasonable likelihood that the psychotic symptoms may be the result of a substance or a general medical condition. In this case, both substance use (e.g., methylphenidate) and a general medical

condition (e.g., narcolepsy) are present, so both Psychotic Disorder Due to a General Medical Condition and Substance-Induced Psychotic Disorder should be considered.

Page 34:   C32 = "+" (delusion of reference)

            C33 = "–" (there is no evidence that the delusion is the direct consequence of Narcolepsy; i.e., delusions are not known to result from Narcolepsy)

Page 35:   C35 = "+" (delusion of reference)

            C36 = "+" (symptoms developed after increasing use of methylphenidate)

            C37 = "+" (not better accounted for by primary psychotic disorder, such as Delusional Disorder, because: 1) the psychotic symptoms did *not* precede the onset of the substance use; 2) the psychotic symptoms are *not* in excess of what you would expect given the amount of methylphenidate being used; and 3) there is no other evidence of an independent non-substance-induced psychotic disorder)

            C38 = "+" (criteria A, B, and C are met—Substance-Induced Psychotic Disorder) Criteria are met in the past month

At this point, you are instructed to return to the disorder being evaluated, in this case back to item C25 on page 32.

Page 32:   C25 = "no" (delusions due to direct physiological effects of a substance)

SCID Diagnosis:
    292.11 Substance-Induced Psychotic Disorder, With Delusions, Current
GAF: 22
    (behavior considerably influenced by delusion—shooting at imaginary intruders)

Homework—Case 7

"Bad Voices"

Carmen Galvez is an attractive, 25-year-old, divorced, Dominican mother of two children, referred to the psychiatric emergency department by a psychiatrist who was treating her in an anxiety disorders clinic. After telling her physician that she heard voices telling her to kill herself and then assuring him that she would not act on the voices, Carmen skipped her next appointment. Her physician called her to say that if she did not voluntarily come to the emergency department for an evaluation, he would send the police for her.

Interviewed in the emergency department by a senior psychiatrist with a group of emergency department psychiatric residents, Ms. Galvez was at times angry and insistent that she did not like to talk about her problems and that the psychiatrists would not believe her or help her anyway. This attitude alternated with flirtatious and seductive behavior.

Ms. Galvez first saw a psychiatrist 7 years previously, after the birth of her first child. At that time, she began to hear a voice telling her that she was a bad person and that she should kill herself. She would not say exactly what it told her to do, but she reportedly drank nail polish remover in a suicide attempt. At that time, she remained in the emergency department for 2 days and received an unknown medication that reportedly helped quiet the voices. She did not return for an outpatient appointment after discharge and continued having intermittent periods of auditory hallucinations over the next 7 years with some periods lasting for months at a time. For example, often when she was near a window, a voice would tell her to jump out, and when she walked near traffic, it would tell her to walk in front of a car.

She reports that she continued to function well after that first episode, finishing high school and raising her children. About 2 months ago, she began to have trouble sleeping and felt "nervous." It was at this time that she responded to an ad for the anxiety clinic. She was evaluated and given Haldol, an antipsychotic. She claims that there was no change in the voices at that time, and only the insomnia and anxiety were new. She specifically denied depressed mood or anhedonia or any change in her appetite but did report that she was more tearful and lonely, and sometimes ruminated about "bad things," such as her father's attempted rape of her at age 14. Despite these symptoms, she continued working more than full-time as a salesperson in a department store.

Ms. Galvez says she did not keep her follow-up appointment at the anxiety clinic because the Haldol was making her stiff and nauseous and was not helping her symptoms. She denies wanting to kill herself, and cited how hard she was working to raise her children as evidence that she would not "leave them that way." She did not understand why her behavior had alarmed her psychiatrist.

Ms. Galvez denied alcohol or drug use, and a toxicology screen for various drugs was negative. Physical examination and routine laboratory tests were also normal. She had stopped the Haldol on her own 2 days before the interview.

Following the interview, there was disagreement among the staff about whether to let the patient leave. It was finally decided to keep her overnight, until her mother could be seen the following day. When told she was to stay in the emergency department, she replied angrily, yet somewhat coyly: "Go ahead. You'll have to let me out sooner or later, but I don't have to talk to you if I don't want to."

When the mother was interviewed the following morning, she said she did not see a recent change in her daughter. She did not feel that Carmen would hurt herself but agreed to stay with her for a few days and make sure she went for follow-up appointments. In the family meeting, Carmen complained that her mother was unresponsive and did not help her enough. However, she again denied depression and said she enjoyed her job and her children. About the voices, she said that over time she had learned how to ignore them and that they did not bother her as much as they had at first. She agreed to outpatient treatment provided the therapist was a female.

SCID Coding for "Bad Voices"

Module A:

Page 13: A1 =   "–" (denied current depressed mood; no information on past)

A2 =   "–" (denied current anhedonia; no information on past)

Page 15: A16 = "–" (no elevated, expansive, or irritable mood)

Page 21: A45 = "–"

Module B:

Page 26: B1 through B5 = "–" (no delusions)

B6 =   "+" (voices telling her to kill herself)

B7 = "–"

Page 27: B8 through B14 = "–"

Module C:

Page 29: C1 =   "yes" (no documentation of mood episodes)

C2 =   "no" (hallucinations but not of a voice keeping up a running commentary or two or more voices conversing)

Page 32: C21 = "no" (no delusions)

Page 33: C27 = "yes" (hallucinations)

C28 = "no" (duration more than one month)

Page 35: C39 = "+" (psychotic symptoms, not meeting criteria for any specific psychotic disorder) Diagnosis has been present in the past month

---

SCID Diagnosis:
289.9 Psychotic Disorder Not Otherwise Specified
GAF: 39
(some impairment in reality testing—intermittent hallucinations)

Homework—Case 8

"Late Bloomer"

Ms. Fielding is a 35-year-old single, unemployed, college educated, African American woman who was escorted to the emergency department by the mobile crisis team. The team had been contacted by the patient's sister after she failed to persuade Ms. Fielding to visit an outpatient psychiatrist. Her sister was concerned about the patient's increasingly erratic work patterns and, more recently, bizarre behavior since the death of their father 2 years ago. The patient's only prior psychiatric contact had been brief psychotherapy in college.

The patient had not worked since being laid off her job 3 months ago. According to her boyfriend and roommate (both of whom live with her), she became intensely preoccupied with the upstairs neighbors. A few days ago she banged on their front door with an iron for no apparent reason. She told the mobile crisis team that the family upstairs was harassing her by "accessing" her thoughts and then repeating them to her. The crisis team brought her to the emergency department for evaluation of "thought broadcasting." Although she denied having any trouble with her thinking, she conceded that she was feeling "stressed" since losing her job and might benefit from more psychotherapy.

After reading the admission note that described such bizarre symptoms, the emergency department psychiatrists were surprised to encounter a poised, relaxed, and attractive young woman, stylishly dressed and appearing perfectly healthy. She greeted them with a courteous, if somewhat superficial, smile. She related to the physicians with nonchalant respectfulness. When asked why she was there, she ventured a timid shrug and replied, "I was hoping to find out from you!"

Ms. Fielding had been working as a secretary and attributed her job loss to the sluggish economy. She said she was "stressed out" by her unemployment. She denied having any recent mood disturbance and answered "no" to questions about psychotic symptoms, punctuating each query with a polite but incredulous laugh. Wondering if perhaps the crisis team's assessment was of a different patient, the interviewer asked, somewhat apologetically, if the patient ever wondered whether people could read her mind. She replied, "Oh yes, it happens all the time," and described how, on one occasion, she was standing in her kitchen planning dinner in silence, only to hear, moments later, voices of people on the street below reciting the entire menu. She was convinced of the reality of the experience, having verified it by looking out the window and observing them speaking her thoughts aloud.

The patient was distressed not so much by people "accessing" her thoughts as by her inability to exercise control over the process. She believed that most people developed telepathic powers in childhood, while she was a "late bloomer" who had just become aware of her abilities and was currently overwhelmed by them. Although she began having telepathic experiences 2 years ago, they had become almost constant in the 3 months since losing her job. She was troubled most by her upstairs neighbors, who would not only repeat her thoughts, but also bombard her with their own devaluing and critical comments, such as "you're no good" and "you have to leave." They had begun to intrude upon her mercilessly, at all hours of the night and day.

She was convinced that the only solution was for the family to move away. When asked whether she had contemplated other possibilities, she reluctantly admitted that she had spoken to her boyfriend about hiring a hit man to "threaten" or, if need be, "eliminate" the couple. She hoped she would be able to spare their two children, whom she felt were not involved in this invasion of her "mental boundaries." This concern for the children was the only insight she demonstrated into the gravity of her symptoms. She did agree, however, to admit herself voluntarily to the hospital.

SCID Coding for "Late Bloomer"

Module A:

Page 13:   A1 =   "–"; A2 = "–"

Page 15:   A16 =   "–"

Page 21:   A45 =   "–"

Module B:

Page 26:   B1 =   "+" (observed people on the street speaking her thoughts aloud)

B2 =   "+" (neighbors are "harassing" her)

B3 =   "–" (her "telepathic" powers are not grandiose in content)

B4 =   "–"

B5 =   "+" (neighbors "accessing" her thoughts; hearing people on the street repeat what she has thought)

B6 =   "+" (neighbors "bombard her with their own devaluing and critical comments")

B7 =   "–"

Page 27:   B8 through B14 = "–"

Module C:

Page 29:   C1 =   "yes" (no Mood Episodes)

C2 =   "yes" (delusions and hallucinations)

C3 =   "yes" (no Mood Episodes)

C4 =   "no" (psychotic symptoms for only 3 months—giving her the benefit of the doubt that the "telepathic experiences" over 2 years are simply her retrospective reinterpretation of events as a result of her current psychotic state)

Page 30:   C13 =   "yes" (psychotic symptoms for 3 months)

C14 =   "yes" (not due to general medical condition or substance)

C15 =   (criteria B and C are met) Criteria met in the past month

---

SCID Diagnosis:
  295.40 Schizophreniform Disorder, Current
GAF: 23
  (behavior considerably influenced by delusions)

Homework—Case 9

"Radar Messages"

Alice Davis, a 24-year-old copy editor who has recently moved from Colorado to New York, comes to a psychiatrist for help in continuing her treatment with a mood stabilizer, lithium. She describes how, 3 years previously, she was a successful college student in her senior year, doing well academically and enjoying a large circle of friends of both sexes. In the midst of an uneventful period in the first semester, she began to feel depressed; experienced loss of appetite, with a weight loss of about 10 pounds; had both trouble falling asleep and waking up too early; had severe fatigue; felt worthless; and had great difficulty concentrating on her school work.

After about 2 months of these problems, they seemed to go away, but she then began to feel increasingly energetic, requiring only 2 to 5 hours' sleep at night, and to experience her thoughts as "racing." She started to see symbolic meanings in things, especially sexual meanings, and began to suspect that innocent comments on television shows were referring to her. Over the next month, she became increasingly euphoric, irritable, and overtalkative. She started to believe that there was a hole in her head through which radar messages were being sent to her. These messages could control her thoughts or produce emotions of anger, sadness, or the like, that were beyond her control. She also believed that her thoughts could be read by people around her and that alien thoughts from other people were intruding themselves via the radar into her own head. She described hearing voices, which sometimes spoke about her in the third person and at other times ordered her to perform various acts, particularly sexual ones.

Her friends, concerned about Alice's unusual behavior, took her to an emergency department, where she was evaluated and admitted to a psychiatric unit. After a day of observation, Alice was started on an antipsychotic, chlorpromazine, and lithium carbonate. Over the course of about 3 weeks, she experienced a fairly rapid reduction in all of the symptoms that had brought her to the hospital. The chlorpromazine was gradually reduced and then discontinued. She was maintained thereafter on lithium carbonate alone. At the time of her discharge, after 6 weeks of hospitalization, she was exhibiting none of the symptoms reported on admission, but she was noted to be experiencing some mild hypersomnia, sleeping about 10 hours a night, and loss of appetite and some feeling of being "slowed down," which was worse in the mornings. She was discharged to live with some friends.

Approximately 8 months after her discharge, Alice was taken off lithium carbonate by the psychiatrist in the college mental health clinic. She continued to do fairly well for the next few months but then began to experience a gradual reappearance of symptoms similar to those that had necessitated her hospitalization. The symptoms worsened, and after 2 weeks she was readmitted to the hospital with almost the identical symptoms that she had had when first admitted.

Alice responded in days to chlorpromazine and lithium, and once again the chlorpromazine was gradually discontinued, leaving her on lithium alone. As with the first hospitalization, at the time of her discharge, a little more than a year ago, she again displayed some hypersomnia, loss of appetite, and the feeling of being "slowed down." For the past year, while continuing to take lithium, she has been symptom free and functioning fairly well, getting a job in publishing and recently moving to New York to advance her career.

Alice's father, when in his 40s, had had a severe episode of depression, characterized by hypersomnia, anorexia, profound psychomotor retardation, and suicidal ideation. Her paternal grandmother had committed suicide during what also appeared to be a depressive episode.

NATIONAL UNIVERSITY LIBRARY ORANGE COUNTY

SCID Coding for "Radar Messages"

Module A:

Page 13: A1 = "+" (3 years ago, began to feel depressed)
A2 = "−"
A3 = "+" (loss of appetite; 10-pound weight loss)
A4 = "+" (trouble falling asleep; waking up too early)
A5 = "−"

Page 14: A6 = "+" (severe fatigue)
A7 = "+" (feelings of worthlessness)
A8 = "+" (difficulty concentrating)
A9 = "−"
A10 = "+"(six A symptoms "+")
A11 = "+" (clinically significant)
A12 = "+" (not due to general medical condition or substance)

Page 15: A13 = "+" (not due to simple bereavement)
A14 = "+" (criteria A, C, D, and E are "+") Criteria have not been met in the past month
A15 = one past Major Depressive Episode
A16 = "+" (3 years ago, became increasingly euphoric and irritable)
A17 = "+" (hospitalized)
A18 = "−"

Page 16: A19 = "+" (required only 3–5 hours of sleep a night)
A20 = "+" (overtalkative)
A21 = "+" (began to experience her thoughts as "racing")
A22 through A24 = "−"
A25 = "+" (three symptoms coded "+")

Page 17: A26 = "+" (hospitalized)
A27 = "+" (not due to a general medical condition or substance)
A28 = "+" (criteria A, C, D, and E are "+") Criteria have not been met in the past month
A29 = two past Manic Episodes

Module B:

Page 26: B1 = "+" (innocent comments on television shows were referring to her)
B2 = "−" (no clear malevolent intent of radar messages)
B3 = "−"
B4 = "+" ("hole in her head")
B5 = "+" (radar messages . . . could control her thoughts; believed her thoughts could be read by other people around her)
B6 = "+" (voices)
B7 = "−"

Page 27: B8 through B14 "−"

Module C:

Page 29: C1 = "no" (psychotic symptoms occur only during Manic Episodes)

Page 36: D1 = "yes" (Manic Episodes)
D2 = "yes" (not due to general medical condition or substance)
D3 = "yes" (not better accounted for by another psychotic disorder)
D4 = 296.46 Bipolar I Disorder, Most Recent Episode Manic, In Full Remission

---

SCID Diagnosis:
296.46 Bipolar I Disorder, Most Recent Episode Manic, In Full Remission
GAF: (Current) 75
(no more than slight impairment in functioning)
